the foot
book

Date: 10/26/11

A Johns Hopkins Press Health Book

the foot *book*

A Complete Guide to Healthy Feet

Jonathan D. Rose, D.P.M.
and Vincent J. Martorana, D.P.M.

The Johns Hopkins University Press
BALTIMORE

Note to the Reader. This book is not meant to substitute for medical care, and treatment should not be based solely on its contents. Instead, treatment must be developed in a dialogue between the individual and his or her physician. Our book has been written to help with that dialogue. At-risk patients, such as people with diabetes or peripheral vascular disease, should never engage in the self-care remedies that are described in this book.

The authors acknowledge the assistance of Bruce Beacham, M.D., F.A.C.P., F.A.A.D., who helpfully reviewed chapter 6 for them.

© 2011 The Johns Hopkins University Press
All rights reserved. Published 2011
Printed in the United States of America on acid-free paper
9 8 7 6 5 4 3 2 1

The Johns Hopkins University Press
2715 North Charles Street
Baltimore, Maryland 21218-4363
www.press.jhu.edu

Library of Congress Cataloging-in-Publication Data

Rose, Jonathan D.
  The foot book : a complete guide to healthy feet / Jonathan D. Rose and Vincent J. Martorana.
    p. cm.
Includes index.
ISBN-13: 978-1-4214-0129-4 (hardcover : alk. paper)
ISBN-13: 978-1-4214-0130-0 (pbk. : alk. paper)
ISBN-10: 1-4214-0129-0 (hardcover : alk. paper)
ISBN-10: 1-4214-0130-4 (pbk. : alk. paper)
  1. Foot—Care and hygiene. I. Martorana, Vincent J. II. Title.
RD563.R587 2011
617.5'85—dc22   2010049757

A catalog record for this book is available from the British Library.

Special discounts are available for bulk purchases of this book. For more information, please contact Special Sales at 410-516-6936 or specialsales@press.jhu.edu.

The Johns Hopkins University Press uses environmentally friendly book materials, including recycled text paper that is composed of at least 30 percent post-consumer waste, whenever possible.

Contents

better appreciation of your feet and helpful information about the possible causes and available treatments for whatever ails them. This book does not cover every single foot and ankle condition, but we have included all those that we regularly see in our practices. We don't mean for the book to replace your physician, nor for it to be a treatment guide in place of consulting a podiatrist. Rather, we intend for readers to use it to gather information before going to a podiatrist or to learn more after receiving a diagnosis. Thus, this book is for people who have or think they may have a foot or ankle problem, as well as for family members of patients and for parents who are concerned about possible problems in their child's feet or way of walking.

This book is in three parts. Part I introduces the development and structure of the foot, various terms used to describe foot positions and movements, and the mechanisms behind how we walk. We discuss basic personal foot care and the podiatry profession in terms of whom you might see for a foot or ankle problem, how to prepare for an appointment, and what types of examinations and tests you can expect. We also provide an overview of shoes and how to choose properly fitting footwear.

Part II consists of nine chapters, each of which discusses foot disorders related to a different part of the foot, such as the toes, toenails, or heel, or to a particular structure within the foot, such as the nerves, joints, or tendons. Every chapter describes various disorders and conditions, and for each we explain the causes, symptoms, diagnosis, and treatment options.

Part III focuses on people with special foot needs, including children, sports enthusiasts, and people with diabetes. The final chapter discusses orthotics, which include custom-molded arch supports, braces, and other devices commonly used to help support and realign feet. At the end of the book is a resources section listing associations and websites that provide additional reliable information.

With the exception of the figure on page 10, the illustrations that appear in the book were drawn by Dr. Martorana and the photographs are from Dr. Martorana's personal collection. Greg Nicholl at the Johns Hopkins University Press assisted with the final preparation of the illustrations.

We hope that this book is helpful as one of the steps you take in learning more about your remarkable feet.

Part One
Introduction

Chapter 1

A Guide to the Foot and How We Walk

MOST OF US DON'T remember a time when we couldn't walk. As infants, we progressed from lying to sitting, crawling to standing, and then to walking—or for some babies, running—long before our first memories took root. When babies take their first staggering steps, they begin their practice of a complex task that involves balance and coordination, muscles and joints, legs and feet. The process of walking is a basic, everyday activity for many people, and, with the obvious exception of those who have mobility difficulties, most people take their ability to walk entirely for granted. They also take for granted the remarkable part of the human body that bears the brunt of a walker's weight and contributes so much to walking: the foot.

As with many aspects of our health, people don't usually think much about their feet until a foot disorder or foot injury causes them pain or difficulty walking. Foot health is extremely valuable to overall body health, and the feet have much to tell as indicators of potential health problems. We would all do well to put up our feet and learn about keeping them healthy.

A first step in understanding more about foot health, foot disorders, and foot injuries is to know a little about the development and anatomy of the foot, as well as the range of movement in a normal foot and ankle.

In Utero and in Childhood: Foot Development

As a baby develops in the womb, a normal series of changes occurs, some of which continue after birth and through the childhood years, and some even to adulthood. In the fetal position, the hips are bent and turned out, as are the knees. The legs are bowed. The normal outward twist from the knee to the ankle, which exists in the adult leg, is absent. The foot itself is often C-shaped (known as *adductus*), the soles of the feet face each other, and the arch is not yet formed.

These shapes and positions aren't exactly favorable for walking on two feet (the activity called *bipedal locomotion*). However, as the infant develops, many torsional (twisting) changes occur. The hip rotates inward as the thigh twists outward, bringing the knee to a forward-facing position. The bowlegged appearance becomes less pronounced and then progresses to knock-kneed before appearing straight. This cycle repeats several times as a child grows and develops, not completing until approximately age 18. An outward twist develops from the knee to the ankle such that by 1½ to 3 years of age, there is a 15-degree outward position in the ankle bones compared with the upper leg bone (tibia). The foot de-rotates so that the soles are perpendicular to the legs within the first several months of life, and the arch begins to form by 3 to 3½ years of age.

Problems develop if growth development stops prematurely or continues beyond what's considered normal development. The result is an altered limb and foot position, which may create abnormal forces on the foot or prevent its normal function. Developmental deformities can occur to varying degrees. In mild cases, the body can compensate, and the variation may not even be identified. More often, there are moderate alterations that may not have an effect for many years. With time, however, the repetitive use of the limb under abnormal alignment takes its toll. Severe deformities are easily recognized at birth and are medically addressed when the treatment can be most helpful.

Clearly, the group with moderate alterations can be of greatest concern because they are less likely to be identified and treated at the appropriate stage in a child's development. These conditions involve variations in alignment, such as the sole of the foot facing excessively inward or outward (known medically as varus or valgus), the foot itself moving into an in-toe (pigeon-toed) or out-toe position, or muscles in the leg pulling the foot upward or allowing it to be too floppy. These conditions are discussed in detail in later chapters.

Anatomy of the Adult Foot

The foot consists of twenty-eight bones—about a quarter of all the bones in the human body are in both feet. The foot's bones are easiest to picture by looking down at the top of the foot, as in figure 1.1. In this view, you see the three sections of the foot: the forefoot, the midfoot, and the hindfoot. The forefoot includes the toes, each of which has two or three *phalanx* bones (collectively they are *phalanges*), and the *metatarsals*, the long bones attached to the toes. The big toe (the *hallux*) has two phalanx bones and one *interphalangeal joint*, and the other four toes each have three phalanx bones

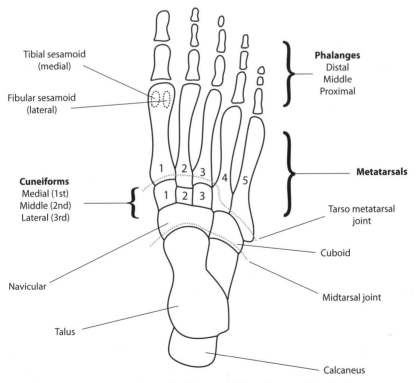

Figure 1.1. The bones in the foot and ankle, viewed from the top (right foot).

and two interphalangeal joints. The phalanx bones are named in sequence, with the nearest to the foot called the proximal, then middle, then distal. The interphalangeal joints are also labeled proximal and distal. The toes join to the metatarsals at the *metatarsophalangeal joints*, which are at the ball of the foot. Below the head of the first metatarsal are two small bones called *sesamoids*.

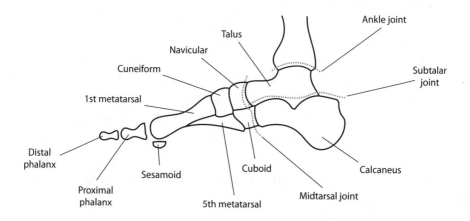

Figure 1.2. The bones in the foot and ankle, viewed from the side (right foot).

The midfoot has five tarsal bones of different shapes and sizes. This part of the foot forms the foot's arch, seen in the side view in figure 1.2, and acts like a stress, or shock, absorber. The hindfoot has two bones, the ankle bone (*talus*) and the heel bone (*calcaneus*), and three joints. The ankle bone connects to the two long lower leg bones (the tibia and fibula) by the *ankle joint*, which is a hinge joint that gives the foot its ability to move up and down. The heel bone, the largest in the foot, connects to the ankle bone at the *subtalar joint*. The third joint in the hindfoot is the *midtarsal joint*, which actually consists of two joints: the *calcaneocuboid*, which joins the calcaneus bone to the cuboid bone, and the *talonavicular*, which joins the talus bone to the *navicular* bone. This midtarsal joint allows the midfoot to turn inward or outward relative to the hindfoot. The hindfoot's joints are seen in the side view in figure 1.2 and also in the view looking at the back of the heel in figure 1.3.

The many joints in the foot and ankle provide flexibility and allow motion wherever bones meet. Joints consist of four types of tissue: cartilage, capsule, ligament, and tendon. *Cartilage* is a tough, wear-resistant tissue that covers the ends of bones in joints and provides protection and cushioning for bones while the joint moves. Its smooth surface allows bones to glide over one another with minimal friction. Most of us are familiar with cartilage as the tissue that gives flexibility to our ears and nose, although joint cartilage is a specialized type that is much harder than the cartilage found in the ears and nose.

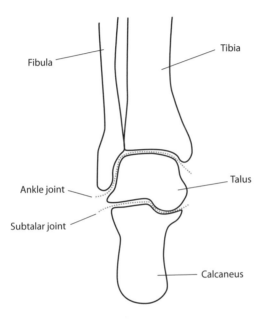

Figure 1.3. The bones in the foot and ankle, viewed from the back (left foot).

Capsule is a soft tissue that forms a structure to encase and support joints. Think of capsule tissue as a form-fitting envelope around a joint. The envelope is lined with a membrane that secretes a fluid to lubricate the joint and reduce friction. *Ligaments* are bundles of fibers that connect one bone to another, hold tendons in place, and help to stabilize joints. The longest ligament in the foot is the *plantar fascia,* which starts at the bottom of the heel and runs underneath the foot to insert into the base of each toe. The plantar fascia contributes to the support, stress absorption, and stability of the foot's arch.

Tendons are tough bands of tissue that join muscles to the foot's bones and joints. Tendons help a joint to move. The largest and strongest tendon is the *Achilles tendon,* which connects the calf muscles to the back of the heel. When a person walks, the Achilles tendon elevates the heel from the ground and contributes to the downward motion of the front of the foot. This tendon's strength enables people to run, jump, and stand on tiptoes. Other tendons in the foot include the *extensor tendons,* on the tops of the toes to pull the toes up, and the *flexor tendons,* on the bottoms of the toes to pull the toes down. The big toe has its own flexor and extensor tendons, so it can move separately, while the four smaller toes share one muscle with four extensor tendon slips, or branches off the main tendon. When the muscle contracts, all four toes extend upward together. Similarly, these toes share a flexor muscle and tendon. The *tibial tendons* and *peroneal tendons* play an important role in stabilizing the foot during walking. The tibial tendons help to move the foot inward toward the midline of the body, while the peroneal tendons help to move the foot outward, away from the midline of the body.

Muscles and tendons both give the foot its shape and enable it to move. The foot's main muscles allow it to move up and down and in and out, help support the foot's arch, lift and curl the toes, and give the toes grip on the ground.

The Mobile Foot: Movements and Positions of the Foot

As you read, lift one foot and move it up and down, left to right, and in circles. If your foot is fairly healthy, you likely can move it into many different positions. The later chapters in this book describe foot disorders and conditions using terms to describe the movements and positions of the foot. Therefore, we define these terms here, for you to use as a reference.

A neutral foot has the body's weight centered over it, with the foot and kneecap directed straight forward. If the foot moves, it leaves its neutral position. The forefoot can move in relation to the midfoot or hindfoot, and the hindfoot can move in relation to the leg. The movements a foot can make are side to side, up and down, and in and out. Each movement has a technical term. Side-to-side movement (figure 1.4) is called

- *adduction* when the foot moves toward the midline of the body. For example, a right foot moves to the left.
- *abduction* when the foot moves away from the midline of the body. For example, a right foot moves to the right.

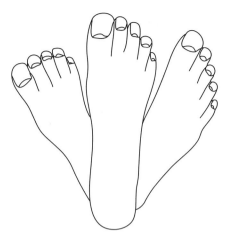

Figure 1.4. From left to right, the foot is adducted, neutral, and abducted.

Up and down movement (figure 1.5) is called

- *dorsiflexion* when the ankle bends to bring the top of the foot up toward the shin. (*Dorsal* refers to the top of the foot.)
- *plantarflexion* when the ankle bends to take the sole of the foot down so that the toes point at the ground. (*Plantar* refers to the bottom or sole of the foot.)

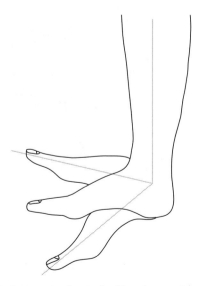

Figure 1.5. From top to bottom, the foot is dorsiflexed, neutral, and plantarflexed.

What Is the Body's Midline?

Draw an imaginary vertical line through the head and core of the body and between the legs: This is called the *midline* of the body. Positions and movements of body parts, such as the foot, are described as orienting toward or away from the midline.

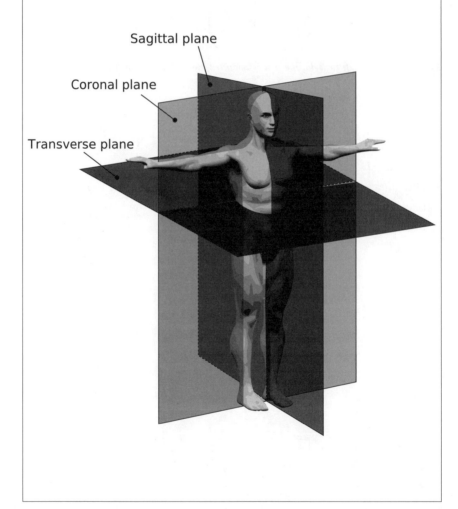

In and out movement (figure 1.6) is called

- *inversion* (varus) when the sole of the foot turns inward to face toward the midline of the body. In other words, the body's weight rolls onto the outer edge.
- *eversion* (valgus) when the sole of the foot turns outward to face away from the midline of the body. In other words, the body's weight rolls onto the inner edge, or arch.

If a foot moves in one of these ways and permanently assumes that position, the foot is in an adductus or abductus position, a dorsiflexed or plantarflexed position, or a varus (inverted) or valgus (everted) position. (The suffix *-us* means a fixed position.)

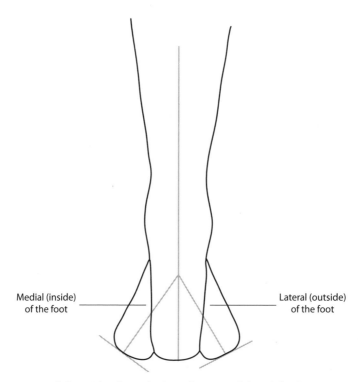

Medial (inside) of the foot   Lateral (outside) of the foot

Figure 1.6. From left to right, this right foot when viewed from behind is varus (inverted), neutral, and valgus (everted).

A foot can make each of the side to side, up and down, and in and out movements separately—one at a time—or a foot can do all three at once, as shown in figure 1.7.

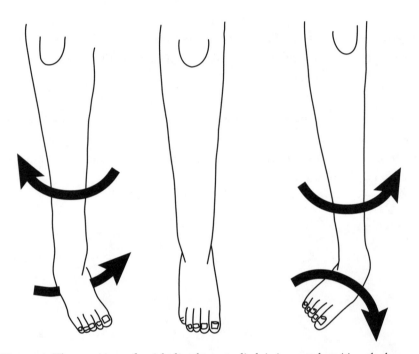

Figure 1.7. Three positions of a right leg: the center limb is in neutral position; the knee-cap and the foot are both directed straight forward. The limb on the left has a supinated foot (adducted, plantarflexed, and inverted) and the leg is externally rotated. The limb on the right has a pronated foot (abducted, dorsiflexed, and everted) and the leg is internally rotated.

- *Supination* describes a foot that simultaneously adducts, plantarflexes, and inverts. Therefore, the foot moves toward the midline, the toes point down, and the weight rolls onto the outer edge so that the sole faces the midline. At the same time, the leg rotates outward.
- *Pronation* describes a foot that simultaneously abducts, dorsiflexes, and everts. Therefore, the foot moves away from the midline, the toes come up toward the shin, and the weight rolls onto the inner edge so that the sole faces away from the midline. At the same time, the leg rotates inward.

A foot that permanently assumes a supinated or pronated position places undue stress on some of the foot's joints. However, supination and pronation are also movements that the foot makes naturally when a person walks.

What Is a "Normal" Foot?

Most of this book discusses problems and abnormalities with the foot. To grasp fully how these problems and abnormalities affect us, it's helpful to understand what constitutes a normal foot. Of course, we must keep in mind that very few people have the "ideal" normal foot, but in general a normal foot should meet seven criteria:

1. Viewed from behind, the heel should be in line with the leg. (The hindfoot should not be in a varus or valgus position.)
2. Viewed from behind, the forefoot should be in line with the hindfoot. (The forefoot should not be in a varus or valgus position.)
3. Viewed from above, the forefoot should be in line with the hindfoot. (The forefoot should not be in an adductus or abductus position.)
4. Viewed from the side, the forefoot should not be lower or higher than the hindfoot, nor the foot lower or higher than the leg. (The forefoot and foot should not be in a plantarflexed or dorsiflexed position.)
5. The leg should not restrict the foot in any of its movements. The leg should not be knock-kneed or bowlegged, which would force the foot in or out.
6. The leg should not be twisted inward or outward, which would force the foot to be in-toe (pigeon-toed) or out-toe.
7. The leg should not restrict upward or downward movement of the foot. The foot should be able to bend upward (dorsiflex) by at least 10 degrees when the knee is straight and the subtalar joint (between the talus and calcaneus bones) is in a neutral position. A tight calf muscle will not allow the foot to bend upward.

All these criteria for a normal foot have to do with alignment. Good alignment is necessary if we expect our feet to support our weight and let us walk and run and do all kinds of other activities without causing us pain. However, the criteria indicate an ideal normal foot. In reality, many feet don't completely meet all the criteria for normalcy, yet a person can be symptom-free and have no walking or running restrictions, because the body is able to compensate for mild to moderate variations in alignment.

Going for a Walk: How We Use Our Feet

When you walk, your legs and feet repeatedly go through a range of positions in the walking, or gait, cycle. The *gait cycle* consists of two phases: The *stance phase* occurs when the foot is in contact with the ground, for about 60 percent of the cycle, and the *swing phase* occurs when the foot is off the ground, for about 40 percent of the cycle. During the stance phase, the foot moves through three basic positions—pronated, neutral, and supinated—each at a precise moment. Understanding when and why the foot assumes each position will help you appreciate the impact that poor mechanics can have on the foot as well as on the limb and body above.

A pronated foot has *unlocked*, or loose, joints, a critical attribute for initial contact with a walking surface, because it allows the foot to adjust to irregularities in the terrain. It also allows the foot to absorb and dissipate shock. Pronation, as described earlier and shown in figure 1.7, is the motion that includes lowering or depressing the arch; everting, or outward tilting of the heel; and abduction, or outward movement of the forefoot relative to the hindfoot. As the foot undergoes these changes, the leg rotates inward.

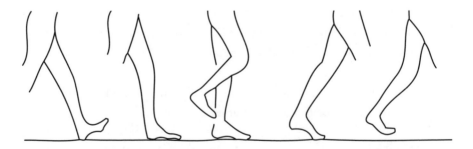

Figure 1.8. Stance phase of the gait cycle, from left to right: heel contact, forefoot contact, midstance, heel off, toe off.

A neutral foot has evenly aligned joints and the heel is vertical and in line with the leg above when viewed from behind. In this position, the muscles are at their *resting length*, the length at which they are physiologically most efficient at providing their function of support and locomotion.

The supinated foot has *locked* joints, which allow the foot to be a rigid lever upon which the muscles contract to propel the body forward. The supinated foot is a very poor shock absorber. Supination is the motion that includes elevating, or raising of the arch; inverting, or inward tilting of the heel; and adduction, or inward movement of the forefoot relative to the hindfoot. At the same time, the leg rotates outward.

Another helpful concept when discussing the gait cycle is the distance between the heel of each foot. When a person is standing, this distance is called the *base of stance* and is measured from center to center of each heel. The average base of stance is 6 to 8 inches, which allows a wide enough base to provide stability. A bowlegged individual has a narrower base, perhaps only 2 to 3 inches, while a knock-kneed individual has a wider base of 10 to 12 inches or more. A wider or narrower base of stance can dramatically affect the foot's function. For example, a knock-kneed position places greater pressure on the inside (medial side) of the foot, which makes it more difficult for the foot to resupinate (elevate the arch) and forces it to function in a pronated position.

When walking, the heel-to-heel distance is measured in the same way and is called the *base of gait*. The base of gait is narrower than the base of stance, because when a person walks, the supporting limb must come closer to the center of the body to prevent the walker from falling over. The average base of gait when walking is 2 inches, and when running, it is close to zero. When a person is running, only one foot touches the ground at a time, so this stance-phase foot must be very close to the midline of the body.

As a person walks, the foot is at a slight angle, either inward or outward from the midline of the body, called the *angle of gait*. A normal angle is approximately 5 degrees outward. An in-toe or out-toe gait can be caused by deviations in the alignment or development of parts of the foot, ankle, leg, or even hip. Excessive in-toe (adductus) or out-toe (abductus) positions place abnormal forces on the foot.

Phases of the Gait Cycle

Of the two gait cycle phases—stance and swing—we concentrate most on the stance phase, because this is when the foot is in contact with the ground and goes through a variety of positions. During the stance phase, faulty bio-mechanics have their most harmful effects on the foot, which we discuss in more detail in chapter 4.

Stance phase consists of five stages: heel contact, forefoot contact, mid-stance, heel off, and toe off, shown in figure 1.8. Stance phase begins as the heel contacts the ground. Just as swing phase is coming to an end, the hip is extended, the knee is extended, the ankle is dorsiflexed, and the foot is supinated. Because of the elevated arch and inverted heel of the supinated position, contact naturally occurs on the heel's outer edge. Both the position of the supinated foot contacting the ground and the narrow base of gait caus-ing the heel to contact on its outer edge explain why it's normal for shoes to get worn down on the outside of the heel. As soon as the heel contacts the ground, the hip and knee momentarily flex (bend) to absorb the shock, and the muscles on the front of the leg begin to slow down the foot's progression to the ground.

With forefoot contact, the foot begins to change from a supinated to a pronated position. As the arch lowers, the heel turns out (everts) and the forefoot turns away (abducts), allowing for further absorption and dissipation of shock. The foot is now maximally pronated, which unlocks the joints and allows the foot to become a mobile adaptor to variable terrain. Momentum carries the opposite hip forward, thereby turning the stance-phase limb out-ward (externally rotating it) and moving the foot toward the neutral position of midstance.

At midstance, all the joints in the stance-phase limb—from the hip joint right down to the interphalangeal joints—are in their neutral position. The body rests directly over the foot, and all the leg and foot muscles are at their resting length, poised to begin the active process of propelling the body for-ward. The body then continues to move forward, so the calf muscles must be supple enough to allow the body to progress past the foot.

In heel off, the ankle bends so that the top of the foot comes closer to the leg (dorsiflexion), while the knee stays straight, and the subtalar joint is in a supinated position. During heel off, the toes bend upward, which tightens the plantar fascia ligament and thereby elevates and strengthens the arch.

As the cycle progresses to toe off, the calf muscles and toe flexors begin to contract to push the foot and toes downward and to propel the body forward.

While one foot contacts the ground and begins stance phase, the opposite foot enters swing phase. The muscles on the front of the leg and the toe extensors are actively firing to lift the foot off the ground while keeping the toes elevated to prevent them from stubbing on the ground as the foot swings through.

Weight shifts across the sole of the foot as the body moves through the gait cycle. The normal progression begins at the outside of the heel when it first contacts the ground. With forefoot contact, the weight travels along the outside of the foot from the heel to the fifth metatarsal head. By midstance, the weight is distributed evenly across the entire sole of the foot, including the heel, the ball of the foot, and the toes. As the heel lifts off the ground, weight shifts to the metatarsal heads and finally, at the toe-off stage, out the end of the big toe.

Chapter 2

Personal Care and Professional Help for Feet

THIS BOOK IS LARGELY about what can go wrong with feet, why foot problems occur, and what can be done to correct or treat the problems. Some foot disorders and conditions happen because of inherited characteristics, pre-existing diseases, or traumatic injury, and they aren't always predictable or easy to prevent. Others, however, can be avoided by following a few basic do's and don'ts of foot care. The first part of this chapter gives some information about personal foot care.

Even with attentive personal foot care, you may need to visit a health professional for a foot problem. If so, it can be helpful to know who the different professionals are and how they can help you. In addition, you can make the most of an appointment by knowing what to expect and by preparing before you go. The second part of this chapter discusses these aspects.

Do's and Don'ts of Personal Foot Care

Taking care of the feet is fairly straightforward for most people and allows them to enjoy good foot health.

Do:
- wash the feet, including between the toes, daily with water and a mild soap.

- thoroughly dry the feet and between the toes after washing them.
- moisturize the feet, but *not* between the toes, after washing them.
- trim the toenails straight across rather than by rounding them.
- inspect the feet regularly (daily if you have diabetes or loss of sensation in your feet) to look for cuts, blisters, signs of infection, dry or scaling skin, embedded objects, changes in moles and other skin marks, and changes in toenails.
- wear shoes that fit properly and that are designed for whatever activity you're doing. Use caution wearing open-toe shoes, sandals, and flip flops: People have been injured wearing such shoes on escalators and elevators.
- alternate shoes from day to day to allow shoes to dry out.
- maintain overall health by eating well, exercising, and avoiding smoking.

Maintaining healthy feet includes a few don'ts as well.

Don't:
- walk barefoot, because of the risk of wounding the feet and getting an infection.
- wear tight or improperly fitting shoes, because they cause problems ranging from blisters to serious damage to the foot's structure and shape.
- share shoes with other people, because of the risk of skin and toenail fungal infections. Shoes lose their inherit support and cushioning as they wear down. Also, shoes wear down according to an individual's structure and function. Sharing a shoe may force a foot into a completely different position. For example, a pronated foot will excessively wear down the inside edge of a shoe, so sharing this shoe with someone who has a supinated foot can have a devastating effect.
- soak the feet in water, because it dries the skin and increases the risk of an open wound becoming infected (from bacteria in the basin or tub). If you really enjoy the relaxation of soaking your feet and you have intact skin—no scaling, cracking, or splitting—soak your feet for no more than ten to fifteen minutes two or three times a week.
- self-treat infections, because they can spread and worsen quickly, even in an otherwise healthy person. If you don't have diabetes, it's fine to self-treat minor cuts and scrapes, but if you have diabetes, poor circulation, or other conditions that have compromised your immune system,

or if there is any question that the area may be infected, seek medical care.

- use over-the-counter cortisone creams or other steroid creams on open wounds or abrasions, because steroids can interfere with the healing of a wound and worsen infection. Steroid creams are better for dermatitis, to treat the rash and resolve the redness and itching.
- ignore moles and other skin marks that are changing in size, shape, appearance, or color or that begin to bleed, because of the possibility that it could be skin cancer. The earlier a skin cancer is caught, the better the outcome.
- ignore pain or other symptoms that persist beyond two or three days, because the body is indicating that something is wrong.

A healthy individual without pain and without any difficulty moving around and participating in activities doesn't need to have a regular foot checkup. However, people with certain health issues, such as diabetes, poor blood circulation, a compromised immune system, and nerve disorders that diminish sensation in the lower leg or foot, should regularly visit a physician for a foot examination, even if they don't have any specific signs or symptoms of foot problems.

Even if you are otherwise healthy, you should go for a medical assessment if you experience or notice:

- persistent pain or swelling in the foot,
- discoloration of the skin or toenails,
- sores that are slow to heal or are not healing on the foot or ankle,
- burning or tingling in the foot,
- pain in the foot or ankle that gets worse with activity,
- a flattening of the foot's arch,
- a mole on the foot or ankle that changes in appearance,
- a lump or bump on the foot or ankle that increases in size or becomes painful,
- a foreign object embedded in the foot or ankle.

Foot Care Professionals: Who Are They?

A health professional who trains to care for people with foot and ankle problems is called a foot and ankle specialist or a podiatrist. For brevity, we generally use the term podiatrist throughout this book. Podiatrists diagnose and treat conditions affecting the foot, ankle, and related structures of the leg. They provide comprehensive medical and, if needed, surgical care for a wide variety of disorders that affect people of all ages.

You may also come across the terms *podiatric physician* and *podiatric surgeon*. There used to be a difference in the training of podiatrists: After they graduated from podiatric medical school, some participated in nonsurgical residencies and others in surgical residencies. However, the training has changed, and now all graduates of podiatric medical school must attend an accredited three-year podiatric surgery residency. Within these three years, the podiatry residents are trained in medical and surgical care for ailments affecting the foot and ankle. There are still some practicing podiatrists who do not perform surgery; these podiatrists are podiatric physicians. The podiatrists who perform surgery are podiatric surgeons as well as podiatric physicians. The American Board of Podiatric Surgery is the certifying board for podiatric surgeons and is recognized by the American Podiatric Medical Association.

If you need to go to a podiatrist, ask your primary care physician or other medical specialist to recommend one. It can also be helpful to talk to other patients about their experiences. Alternatively, contact your local hospital referral line for the names of podiatrists on staff or contact the American Board of Podiatric Surgery for a list of certified podiatric surgeons in your area. If you are considering a surgical solution for your foot or ankle problem, we strongly recommend that you ask whether the podiatrist is certified by the American Board of Podiatric Surgery. The resources section lists contact information for this and other associations.

Like any other physician, podiatrists work with and refer patients to medical professionals in other specialities. We mention a variety of other medical professions in this book, including vascular surgeons (blood and lymph systems), neurologists (nerves and nervous system), rheumatologists (muscles, tendons, and joints, especially arthritis), endocrinologists (pancreas [diabetes], thyroid and other glands, and hormones), oncologists (tumors and cancer),

and dermatologists (skin). We also mention physical therapists, who help
people to restore and improve muscle and joint function, and orthotists and
pedorthists, who make custom braces and shoes.

Be Prepared: What Should You Do before a Podiatry Appointment?

Once you have an appointment with a podiatrist, prepare so that you make
the most of your visit. Always take a complete list of all current medications—
or take the bottles with you. If you have allergies of any sort, bring a list of
them as well. It's helpful for a podiatrist to know what tests you've had before,
such as x-rays, magnetic resonance imaging (MRI), computed tomography
scans, or blood work, and ideally to see the actual films or study results as
well as the written report prepared by the physician who ordered the tests. If
possible, ask doctors you've seen previously to send your patient record to the
podiatrist in advance of your visit. (You will need to sign a release form to
have your record sent.) Last, make sure you have the appropriate paperwork
if your insurance company requires a referral from a primary care provider or
another authorization for patients to be seen by a specialist.

Before you go to your appointment, wash your feet and, though it may
seem obvious, put on clean socks. If you perspire heavily, use a small amount
of powder on your feet. Remove nail polish, especially for initial office visits,
even if the problem you have is not related to the toes or toenails. The doctor
needs to see the condition of the nails because they can often provide a clue
to a diagnosis. Ideally, wear loose pants that can be rolled up to allow the
podiatrist to examine the lower leg. Shorts and skirts also work well, although
women should avoid wearing short skirts, because the position in which a
woman sits to have her feet examined can be awkward for both the patient
and the doctor.

Be prepared to answer a range of questions at your appointment. The podiatrist will want to know what symptoms you've been experiencing and
how long they've been going on, when the problem started, the nature and
specific location of pain, what aggravates the problem or symptoms and
what relieves them, and what, if any, treatment you've attempted. In addition,
the podiatrist needs to know if you've already seen any physicians for the
problem.

You will also be asked to provide the podiatrist with details of your medical and surgical history. Be prepared to answer questions that may seem personal or unrelated to your foot complaint. For example, heel pain can be related to some inflammatory joint conditions, which have symptoms such as pink eye, a burning sensation when urinating, and skin rashes. Answer all questions honestly and accurately so that the podiatrist can make a correct diagnosis and identify the best treatment options. You should also mention if you have any activities or trips scheduled that may have to be considered in the treatment plan. It's a good idea to write things down before you go to the appointment, so you won't forget anything.

Typically, a podiatrist's services are covered by health insurance plans. The only exception is routine cutting of nails and calluses; however, patients with certain conditions, including some nerve and circulatory system disorders, may be eligible for coverage of nail cutting and callus trimming. Medicare covers these services for some people with diabetes, usually only if they have lost normal sensation in the feet or have poor circulation. Most health insurance plans don't cover orthotics, but some do. If orthotics are being considered as part of your treatment plan, contact your insurance company about coverage. Your podiatrist's office staff may also be able to inquire about this on your behalf.

What Can You Expect at a Podiatry Appointment?

A visit to a podiatrist entails the usual things you encounter with any medical professional. First, you will be asked to fill out paperwork with your insurance information, emergency contacts, and medical history. The podiatrist will take a complete medical history from you, including past illnesses and surgeries and current medications. Next, the podiatrist will conduct a physical examination of the foot or ankle, depending on the symptoms you describe. He or she will probably take a look at your shoes and may ask you to walk back and forth in the examining room to evaluate your gait. If necessary, the podiatrist takes x-rays (if the office is set up with x-ray machinery), or orders x-rays or other imaging tests to be done by another provider.

There is a wide range of other tests and examinations that the podiatrist may carry out, again depending on your foot complaint. We briefly describe what is involved in some common tests. Additional tests are described in later chapters if they are typically done to evaluate certain conditions.

A vascular examination assesses the circulatory system. The examiner checks pulses in the foot, looks for redness of the skin, and does a capillary refill test. The capillary refill test determines how quickly blood refills empty capillaries (small blood vessels). The test is done by pressing on the soft pad of a toe until it turns white, then releasing and noting how long it takes for the skin to return to its natural color. It should take less than three seconds.

A neurological examination tests reflexes, the sensation of vibrations made against the skin with a tuning fork, and the sensation from touching different parts of the foot and ankle with a flexible nylon wire called a Semmes-Weinstein monofilament.

A musculoskeletal examination manually tests the strength and function of muscles; assesses misalignments in the foot, ankle, and leg; and examines any bony outgrowths. The exam also tests joints for stiffness and their range of motion.

A dermatologic examination assesses discoloration, warmth, redness, callus formation, moles, and vein abnormalities.

Don't be shy about asking questions and taking notes. The podiatrist is there to find out what is wrong and to make sure you understand the nature of the problem and the prognosis, what may have caused the problem, and what treatment options you have. If you don't understand something, ask for clarification. Find out what you should and should not do to keep the problem from getting worse or from recurring after treatment. For any suggested treatment, find out whether it will affect your ability to work or do your regular daily activities. If the podiatrist recommends taking medication, ask about side effects and possible interactions with other medications you take. If surgery is a possibility, find out whether conservative treatments could be tried first, how successful the surgery usually is, how long the recovery period is, and what's involved in recovery (e.g., wearing a cast, going to physical therapy). When considering any treatment option, particularly surgical treatment, you need to weigh the potential benefits with the risks. The podiatrist can help you understand these, but ultimately the decision to pursue a particular treatment is yours. In making a decision, consider your medical health, age, activity level, and expectations after treatment.

By the end of your appointment with a podiatrist, you should have a better idea of what may be wrong with your foot or ankle. The complete diagnosis may not be made, especially if the podiatrist needs to refer you for a more detailed examination by another specialist or if you need to have x-rays, MRI, or other tests done at a different location. However, many of the conditions discussed in this book, such as ingrown toenails, warts, corns and calluses, and heel pain, can be treated at the first visit to a podiatrist. At the least, treatment is often initiated, and follow-up visits are scheduled to treat the condition until the symptoms resolve.

As a patient, you are entitled to seek a second opinion or to switch to a different medical professional if you want to. We recommend looking for a different podiatrist if you're unhappy with the care you're receiving, if you have communication difficulties with the physician, or if cultural differences might interfere with the patient–physician relationship. If you are having difficulty communicating with the podiatrist's staff, you should discuss this with the doctor. We also recommend seeking a second opinion if you are deciding whether or not to pursue extensive reconstructive foot or ankle surgery. Most experienced physicians welcome a request for a second opinion.

Chapter 3

About Shoes

NEARLY EVERYONE WEARS SHOES of one kind or another. We choose different shoes for different activities, though some people make choices more motivated by fashion than by what their feet really need. What is crucial about a shoe is that it supports, cushions, and protects the foot. Wearing the right shoe for your foot and for the activity you're doing—whether it's standing, walking, running, or anything else—can promote normal foot function and provide needed stability and support. In this chapter, we describe the parts of a shoe, how shoes are designed, how to know if a shoe fits you properly, and a few types of shoes to wear with caution. Some other chapters in the book include specific information about shoes for children (chapter 13), for people who play sports (chapter 14), and for people with diabetes (chapter 15).

Shoe Savvy

Shoes are so much more than simply coverings for the feet. To better appreciate the job your shoes have, first understand the role each part of a shoe—sole, upper, heel, heel counter, toe box, shank, last—plays in enhancing the way your foot works.

The bottom, or sole, of a shoe has three parts: the insole, the outsole, and the midsole. The *insole* is the layer that makes direct contact with the foot in the interior of the shoe. It can often be replaced with a more supportive or accommodative over-the-counter insole or custom-made orthotic. An insole can also be modified to increase cushioning for the foot or take weight off a particular part of the foot.

The *outsole* is the undersurface that makes contact with the ground and provides traction or grip. It may be made of leather, which is common in dress shoes, or of rubber, usually in casual or athletic shoes. The outsole can be modified to relieve pressure and to encourage a more functional gait. Sole modifications that may reduce pressure to the toes and forefoot include a rocker sole, a metatarsal bar, and a steel or carbon fiber plate reinforcement. Wedges can be added to the inside or outside of the outsole to move the foot into a more supinated position (shifting weight toward the outer edge) or pronated position (shifting weight toward the inner edge).

The *midsole*, not surprisingly, is the layer between the insole and the out-sole. It provides cushioning, shock absorption, and stability to the shoe. The midsole should bend or be flexible at the point where the toes meet the foot. The midsole can be modified to strengthen the arch, which helps a foot resist rolling inward (pronation). Also, flares can be added to the sides of the heels to provide increased stability. Modifications to the outsole or midsole usually require a prescription and can be done by an orthotist, pedorthotist, or prosthetist at a specialized shoe store.

The *upper*, or vamp, of a shoe helps to hold the shoe to the foot. For a lace-up shoe, the laces are part of the upper. Ideally, the upper is padded to cushion the top of the foot. Athletic shoes should have a lightweight and breathable upper. For people with toe problems, the upper should be a soft and stretchable material to reduce toe irritation.

The *heel*, the bottom part at the back of the shoe, provides cushioning, stability, and sometimes elevation to the back part of the foot. Heel modifications include cushioning for shock absorption, lifts to compensate for a tight heel cord or shortened limb, and wedges or flares to keep the foot from shifting inward or outward.

The *heel counter*, or heel cup, is the cup-shaped reinforcement that supports the back and sides of the heel. In addition to providing support, the heel counter limits excessive heel motion. All shoes should have a firm to hard heel counter. A shoe with an inadequate heel counter will not be able to withstand the forces of a misaligned foot, causing the shoe to break down, which magnifies the severity of the deformity, as seen in figure 3.1.

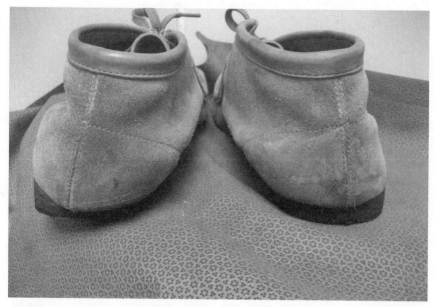

Figure 3.1. The lack of an appropriate heel counter in these shoes has allowed a pronated foot to break them down. A good shoe provides support that controls abnormal forces from the foot.

The *toe box* is the front part of the shoe and may be square, rounded, or pointed. To accommodate toe and forefoot problems, the toe box can be modified by increasing the width and depth of the shoe to make a so-called extra-depth shoe.

The *shank* of the shoe is the section of the sole that connects the heel to the toe box. For most shoes, the shank should be rigid to prevent the shoe from buckling below the arch. The shank is typically made of plastic or steel.

The *last* of the shoe is its overall shape. The last usually curves at the arch to conform to the average person's foot, helping to distinguish the right shoe from the left. The last can be modified, particularly for children, to correct a foot deformity or to maintain a corrected foot in its proper position.

Function over Fashion: Shoe Design

The design of a shoe takes into account all sorts of factors. One particularly important factor is the distance between a person's feet. This distance varies depending on whether a person is standing, walking, or running. The base of stance is the distance between the center of each heel when you stand, and the base of gait is this distance when you walk or run. The base of stance is 6 to 8 inches wide for stability. As you walk and then run, the base of gait gets narrower, because the foot moves closer to the body's midline so that you don't fall over. The average base of gait is 2 inches when walking and close to zero when running.

A shoe designed for normal standing typically has the heel counter mounted perpendicular, or at right angles, to the sole of the shoe because the leg and back of the heel should be in line with each other and perpendicular to the floor. When you walk, the foot contacts the ground in a slightly inverted position. Therefore, a shoe designed for walking has the heel counter mounted at a slight angle to the sole. In a running shoe, the heel counter is mounted at an even greater angle. Note, however, that the angle of the heel counter is not visible from the outside of the shoe. From the outside, the heel counter of all shoes appears to be at right angles to the shoe's sole.

The inverted heel counter of a running shoe is ideal for running straight ahead but not for a sport, such as tennis or basketball, that requires side-to-side movements. In these sports, wearing a shoe designed for forward running makes an athlete more prone to ankle sprains. Therefore, people should buy sport-specific shoes. A cross trainer is a blended shoe that allows for some side-to-side movement while also providing some of the shock absorption required of a running shoe. Additional information about sports shoes is included in chapter 14.

If the Shoe Fits . . .

For both men and women, shoes should be comfortable—right from day one. There is no such thing as a break-in period. If a shoe pinches or rubs or feels too tight, don't buy the shoes. Shoe size and fit vary widely between styles and manufacturers, so keep looking until you find a shoe that properly fits your foot. A proper fit means that the shoe should have an adequate toe box and a low, cushioned heel (half an inch or less). The heel counter should fit snugly, and your foot should not slide around in the shoe. Fit shoes to accommodate your longest and widest foot, and make sure there's a half-thumbnail width between the longest toe and the end of the shoe. The upper shouldn't bulge over the sole of the shoe. Although you should not have to break in shoes, new shoes with stiff soles, such as leather, may not bend easily at the ball of the foot, causing the shoe to slip up and down on the back of the heel. As you wear the shoe, the sole becomes more flexible and the heel slipping diminishes.

Try to shop for new shoes at the end of the day, when your feet are at their largest, since feet swell over the course of the day. Have both feet measured for length and width when you're standing up. Try on shoes while wearing the socks or stockings you intend to wear with them. If possible, wear and walk around in shoes for at least ten minutes in the store to check for comfort before buying them. If you use an orthotic, be sure to wear it while you're trying on new shoes. Before you buy, evaluate the shoes for defects, such as a crooked heel, loosely glued midsole, or a sole that isn't even on a level surface. You shouldn't be able to rock in the shoes when you have them on.

Not All Shoes Are Made Alike

Some shoes do the exact opposite of what shoes should do, causing serious problems rather than supporting and cushioning the foot. High heels, flip flops and sandals, and high-top shoes and boots can all cause problems with your feet and ankles.

We strongly advise that most women not wear high-heeled shoes, especially not routinely, because these shoes encourage foot deformities to develop and can lead to painful symptoms in the ankle, calf, and lower back. However, there are some women whose feet fit extremely well into high heels and who actually do poorly with low heels or flat shoes, for example, women whose feet have very high arches, as in figure 3.2.

Flip flops and many sandals present a wide range of problems for feet. They lack arch support, which can cause pain in various joints and tendons; they don't provide protection from fallen objects; and they expose the top of the foot to the sun, which increases the chance of developing skin cancer. Injuries to the foot can occur by getting a loose sandal caught when getting on and off elevators and escalators, and even by opening a door across the tops of one's own toes. Walking in flip flops requires the toes to grasp the

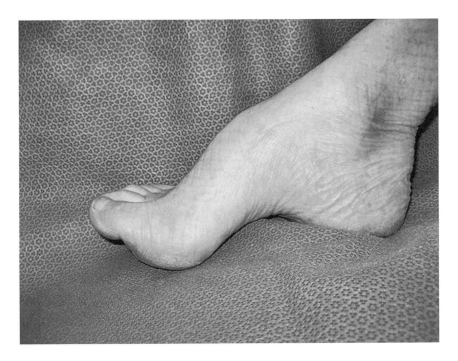

Figure 3.2. A high-arched foot, where the forefoot is much lower than the heel.

shoe for balance and to keep the shoe on, making the toes work more than they do in a shoe with a heel counter. The toes are also more likely to be stubbed. Last, a strap between the big toe and second toe can create an open wound and infection.

High-top shoes or boots can also create a number of problems. If they're too tight, they can irritate nerves close to the skin surface and cause a nerve condition called neuritis. Many Ugg boots, work boots, and western boots have poor arch support and little or no cushioning. For people with a condition known as Haglund's deformity, which is a bony outgrowth at the back of the heel, wearing high-top shoes and boots is painful and can lead to a bursitis. These conditions are discussed in chapter 9.

Part Two

Foot Disorders and Other Problems

Chapter 4

Foot Alignment Problems

THE ONLY CONTACT A CAR has with the road is through the tires on its wheels, so the condition and alignment of the tires and wheels have a profound effect on the car's driving performance. Imagine the quality of a ride in a car with one unaligned wheel. If it's badly out of alignment, the ride will be rough, and the car will probably develop mechanical problems. In the same way, a poorly aligned foot can make walking difficult and even painful, and it can have profound effects on the rest of the body.

Very few people have "ideal" normal feet, but fortunately, the human body compensates for minor variations. Over time, however, even small compensations can take their toll. In this chapter, we describe the most common foot alignment problems, how they affect the foot's function, and treatment options.

Out of Line: Varus and Valgus Abnormalities

When a normal foot is in a neutral position, the forefoot should be in line with the hindfoot, and the hindfoot should be at right angles to the heel. The neutral position is shown in figure 4.1. A variation occurring in either the forefoot or the hindfoot results in a fixed varus or valgus abnormality ("fixed" because without treatment, the foot would be permanently in the abnormal position). In these abnormalities, the sole of the foot—whether it's the sole of the forefoot or of the heel—turns to face inward, or inverts (varus), or turns to face outward, or everts (valgus). Another way to think of these conditions is that a varus foot rolls the body's weight to the outside of the foot, while a valgus foot rolls weight to the inside, or arch, of the foot.

A *hindfoot varus* is diagnosed when the heel is inverted in relation to the leg (figure 4.2). Most people with a hindfoot varus will compensate by pronating the hindfoot (allowing the heel to turn out) to bring the inside of the foot to the ground. Left untreated, this position forces a person to walk on the outside of the foot, which creates problems with shock absorption and strain from uneven weight distribution across the foot.

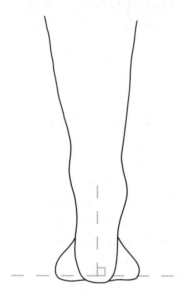

Figure 4.1. Normal relationship of the forefoot to the hindfoot and the hindfoot to the heel in the neutral position (right leg).

Forefoot varus occurs when the forefoot is inverted in relation to the hind-foot (figure 4.3). The foot can't function in this position, so the subtalar joint pronates, or rolls the body's weight to the inside edge, to bring the forefoot to the ground. This pronation of the foot can be even more extreme than with a hindfoot varus, and it can have several long-term effects. A pronated foot is a loose and mobile adaptor to the terrain when walking, and while this is desirable during initial contact with the ground, it doesn't allow for proper support or an efficient lever for the muscles to propel the body forward. In addition, the leg and thigh rotate toward the midline of the body when the foot pronates. Over time, a leg in this rotated position decreases the ability of the kneecap (*patella*) to glide or track smoothly. Poor kneecap tracking may progress to pain at the front of the knee, a condition known as chondromalacia patella, or runner's knee (although people participating in all sorts of activities and sports may experience it). Further up the skeletal system, the muscles that connect the thigh to the pelvis and low back (the *iliopsoas* muscles) may be overworked when the foot is excessively pronated, causing fatigue and cramping that results in low back pain. Also, an excessively pronated foot increases the incidence of abnormalities such as bunions and hammertoes (chapter 8) and tendon injury (chapter 12).

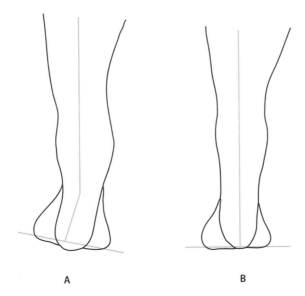

A B

Figure 4.2. A right foot, as seen from behind, showing (A) a hindfoot varus, in which the heel is turned in relative to the leg, and (B) compensation, in which the heel turns out to bring the heel perpendicular to the ground and the front of the foot to the ground.

A *hindfoot valgus* is one in which the heel is turned out, or everted, in relation to the leg (figure 4.4), the position associated with flat or pronated feet. In most instances, the muscles of the leg aren't strong enough to overcome the heel's everted position and invert the foot. When the heel is in an everted position, the foot remains pronated throughout the gait cycle,

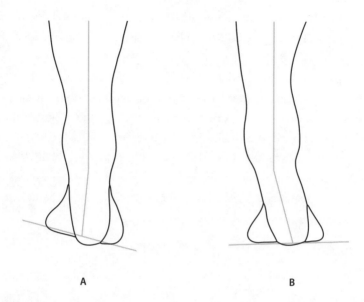

A   B

Figure 4.3. A right foot, as seen from behind, showing (A) a forefoot varus, in which the forefoot is turned in relative to the hindfoot, and (B) compensation, in which the heel turns out in an excessively pronated position.

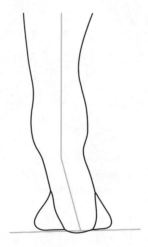

Figure 4.4. A right foot, as seen from behind, showing a hindfoot valgus, in which the heel is turned out relative to the leg. The foot muscles rarely have the strength to compensate, so the foot remains pronated.

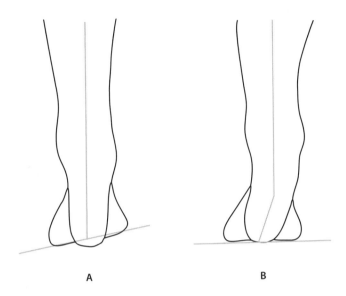

A   B

Figure 4.5. A right foot, as seen from behind, showing (A) a forefoot valgus, in which the forefoot is turned out relative to the hindfoot, and (B) compensation, in which the heel turns in to bring the front of the foot to the ground.

which, as mentioned before, doesn't provide a stable supporting structure or a rigid lever to efficiently propel the body forward. In addition, a person with hindfoot valgus may experience knee or back pain and may also develop conditions like bunions, hammertoes, and tendon injury. Flat feet are discussed in greater detail in chapter 5.

A *forefoot valgus*, in which the forefoot is everted relative to the hindfoot (figure 4.5), is commonly associated with a high-arched (*pes cavus*) foot. This condition typically places an increased load on the first metatarsal, resulting in painful calluses below the first metatarsal and conditions such as sesamoiditis (see chapter 14). The body compensates by inverting the heel (supinating the subtalar joint), which can result in an unstable ankle that's susceptible to ankle sprains (see chapter 14). High-arched feet are discussed in greater detail in chapter 5.

The treatment of varus and valgus conditions aims to reduce pain in the foot and improve the foot's function. Treatment usually begins with conservative measures, typically changing or modifying the shoes you wear, using an orthotic, or having physical therapy. You can also consider surgery, but we don't advise this until conservative measures have been tried without success.

Ankle Bending: Dorsiflexion and Plantarflexion Abnormalities

Bending the ankle to lift the foot toward the front of the leg (dorsiflexion) or lower it away from the leg (plantarflexion) are movements that a normal ankle and foot do easily and painlessly. However, these movements can be restricted for various reasons. The normal range of movement is to be able to dorsiflex the foot by 20 degrees from neutral and plantarflex the foot by 50 degrees. The minimal requirement for walking is to be able to dorsiflex the foot by at least 10 degrees when the knee is straight and the subtalar joint is in a neutral position. When either dorsiflexion or plantarflexion is compromised, a person has difficulty walking with a normal gait and may find running particularly hard to do. Other activities can also be awkward, such as getting the foot onto a car's brake pedal or pushing the gas pedal to the floor.

Toe Walking

When a person can dorsiflex the foot by only a few degrees, or not at all, the condition is referred to as *ankle equinus,* or toe walking. In normal walking, the ankle dorsiflexes to allow the heel to make the first contact with the ground. If the top of the foot can't be brought up in this way, then the toes contact the ground before the rest of the foot, hence the term toe walking.

A common reason for an ankle equinus is tightness in one of the three calf muscles—the medial and lateral gastrocnemius muscles and the soleus muscle—that form the Achilles tendon. Ankle equinus can also be caused by a bone spur, or bony outgrowth, in the front of the ankle. Often, the extra piece of bone is on the upper surface of the talus bone, and it hits the front of the tibia bone when the foot is dorsiflexed. In other cases, the forefoot is plantarflexed in relation to the hindfoot, meaning that the forefoot is lower than the hindfoot (see figure 3.2 in chapter 3). Known as *forefoot equinus*, this foot position requires additional ankle dorsiflexion to lift the forefoot off the ground and prevent the toes from stubbing on the floor during swing phase of the gait cycle.

The body's compensation for an ankle equinus or a forefoot equinus can have devastating consequences for the foot, knees, hips, and lower back. To walk normally and progress beyond midstance, the foot must be able to dorsiflex by at least 10 degrees. If the ankle can't bend to this degree, then something will have to give as momentum drives the body beyond the foot, which is fixed against the nonyielding floor. There are three possible compensations that the body can make:

1. The first, which provides the needed flexibility to walk, is excessive pronation or unlocking of the subtalar and midtarsal joints. This excessive unlocking, combined with the weight of the body above the foot, can be severe enough to cause the foot's arch to collapse. A collapsed arch can result in tendon injury, particularly to the posterior tibial tendon, which can progress to tendon degeneration and eventually tendon rupture (see chapter 12). A collapsed arch also causes excessive wear and tear on the joints, leading to premature osteoarthritis (see chapter 11).
2. The second possible compensation is for the knee to hyperextend to allow the body to pass beyond the foot. The consequence of knee hyperextension is increased strain on the knee joint.
3. The third compensation is for the heel to lift off the ground prematurely to allow the body to pass beyond the foot, an action that results in a bopping gait. This bopping gait may draw unwanted attention, and it can lead to forefoot pain from metatarsalgia (chapter 8) and Achilles tendonitis (chapter 9).

If you go to a podiatrist because of a toe-walking problem, he or she will conduct a physical examination to diagnose the reason for the equinus and to recommend appropriate treatment. The examination entails manually moving your foot up toward the shin with your knee straight and then with your knee bent. This manipulation is done with your foot in a neutral position, then a supinated position, and finally a pronated position. If the podiatrist suspects that a bone is blocking the foot's movement, you will be x-rayed. Treatment for equinus initially involves relieving the symptoms. A shoe with an elevated heel or a heel lift inside it helps to relieve strain on the Achilles tendon. Your symptoms may be treated with nonsteroidal anti-inflammatory drugs (NSAIDs), ice, physical therapy, or immobilization of the foot with a CAM walker (a walking cast that is like a rigid boot). You may also be advised to wear a custom-made orthotic to treat compensatory pronation.

Treating the equinus itself depends on the cause. Most often, you will be encouraged to do flexibility and stretching exercises to stretch the Achilles tendon (see the first box in chapter 9). In severe cases, the Achilles tendon may need to be surgically lengthened. If a bone spur or bony outgrowth is the cause, surgery removes the extra bone.

Spastic Toe Walking

A foot that maintains a rigid downward position is termed a *spastic equinus*, because it results from spasm of the muscles at the back of the leg. Spastic equinus can occur if scar tissue forms after trauma to the ankle joint or if surgical repair of the joint, for example after an ankle fracture, creates scar tissue or a tightening of the joint's capsule tissues. Also, many people with cerebral palsy have spastic equinus, because cerebral palsy affects motor control of the body. With this form of toe walking, the foot's rigid position puts increased pressure on the forefoot, leading to metatarsalgia (chapter 8), calluses (chapter 6), and sometimes ulcers (open wounds). Treatment usually involves wearing special accommodative shoes or a brace and, in some cases, surgery.

Drop Foot

Drop foot is a condition in which the foot, when it's not resting on the ground, is plantarflexed, and the foot's muscles are unable to bring the foot up, not even to a neutral position. With drop foot, it is difficult or impossible to walk without using the thigh muscles (quadriceps) to lift the leg higher so that the foot clears the ground. People with an untreated drop foot tend to drag their toes on the ground as the foot begins the swing phase of the gait cycle, which may cause them to trip or fall. Frustrating and humiliating for most people, this condition can be particularly dangerous for the elderly. A drop foot usually occurs because of weak dorsiflexor muscles, which typically result from neurological disorders or nerve entrapments (see chapter 10). Treatments for drop foot include changing or modifying your shoes or using a brace. Surgery to transfer tendons within the foot is also a possibility, and in some cases, the ankle can be surgically immobilized or fused.

In and Out: Adduction and Abduction Abnormalities

A person whose foot, or a part of whose foot, moves either toward or away from the midline of the body stands in an in-toe or an out-toe position. An in-toe position is called adductus, and an out-toe position is called abductus. The cause of these abnormalities can originate from within the foot or from the limb above.

When an in-toeing problem occurs from within the foot, it is termed a *metatarsus adductus*. In this condition, the forefoot deviates toward the midline of the body in relation to the midfoot and hindfoot (when viewed from above or below). The result is a C-shaped foot, as shown in figure 4.6. Often, metatarsus adductus forces the base of the fifth metatarsal to push out from the outside of the foot. This shifting can cause bursitis (inflammation of a bursa, or sac, between a tendon and a bone) or tendonitis (inflammation of a tendon) of the *peroneus brevis tendon*, the tendon that joins to the base of the fifth metatarsal. Metatarsus adductus can result in painful calluses and may even lead to foot ulcers in patients with diabetes or poor circulation. Sometimes, the body tries to compensate by pronating the subtalar joint in an attempt to bring the front of the foot back into alignment. Pronation can lead to hammertoes, bunions, and tendon injury. In addition, osteoarthritis can occur at the tarsometatarsal joint (see chapter 11).

Treatment alternatives include using protective pads behind and below (not directly on) the bony prominence to reduce pressure, taking NSAIDs, using ice on an area with bursitis or tendonitis, and trimming a callus, if present. In addition, you can wear an orthotic to accommodate the bony prominence and reduce pressure from your shoes or from walking on the foot. Physical therapy helps to reduce inflammation. Cortisone can also be used to decrease inflammation but should be a treatment of last resort, just short of surgery, because cortisone can further weaken a chronically inflamed tendon and cause it to rupture, a complication that itself requires surgery. Rarely is it necessary for an adult to undergo surgery to correct metatarsus adductus, although surgical planing (shaving) of the prominent bone at the

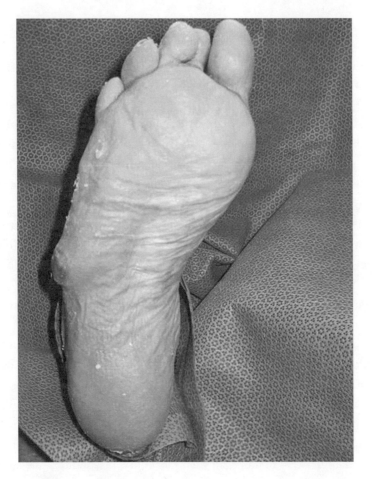

Figure 4.6. Metatarsus adductus showing a typical callus at the base of the fifth metatarsal.

fifth metatarsal base with reattachment of the tendon is an option for un-manageable pain. Treatment for metatarsus adductus in infants is addressed in chapter 13.

The foot can also be affected by abnormal influences from the limb above, such as internal or external rotation, also resulting in an in-toe or out-toe position. Rotations that occur in the hip, thigh, and leg can cause an in-toe or out-toe gait as well. In-toe and out-toe positions due to the limb above usu-ally develop during fetal gestation. We discuss these abnormalities in chapter 13 as well.

Long and Short: Differences in Limb Length

Although the human body is built with two halves that look like mirror images, they rarely are. Many people have asymmetrical legs, so that one leg is or appears to be longer than the other. Differences in limb length can be a structural discrepancy or a functional discrepancy. A structural discrepancy is due to a true difference in the length of the bones from one side of the body to the other. A structural discrepancy can result from a genetic disorder, a congenital condition (occurring in the womb, but not genetic), or premature closing of a bone's growth plate because of infection, surgery, bone fracture, or tumor. A functional discrepancy can be due to any number of things, such as asymmetry of arch height from one foot to the other, a dislocated hip, or a curved spine (scoliosis). For example, a person with a flat foot on only one side will experience a functional limb length discrepancy. This type of discrepancy can have profound effects on the entire body as the person compensates for the difference.

When the body compensates for a difference in leg length, the goal, though not a conscious one, is to bring the eyes to a plane parallel to the floor. Sometimes, the longer limb pronates, or shifts the body's weight to the inside of the foot, as a means of shortening the leg. Other times, the foot on the shorter side will supinate, or shift weight to the outer margin, thereby raising the arch and effectively lengthening the leg. Typically, the pelvis tilts down on the shorter side, and the lower spine then curves in the opposite direction. For example, if the left leg is shorter, the pelvis tilts down on the left side and the lower spine curves to the right. These pelvic and spinal compensations may progress to the point that the upper spine and shoulders tilt as well. If the spine can't adjust enough to accommodate for the difference in leg length, the neck may tilt to bring the eyes level. All of these compensations by the body, no matter how subtle, can affect the functioning of bones, joints, muscles, ligaments, and nerves. Symptoms can range from pain, cramping, and spasms to fatigue affecting the foot, leg, knee, hip, low back, and neck.

The treatment of a limb length discrepancy depends on the reason for the different lengths and the amount by which the legs differ. If you have a minimal structural discrepancy, you may need only a simple heel raise or lift.

With a difference less than a quarter to three-eighths of an inch, the adjustment can be made within your shoe in the form of a removable heel lift. For a greater difference, a portion of the correction can be made within your shoe and the remainder by an addition to the outside of the heel or sole of the shoe. For functional discrepancies due to variations in the height of the arch, a combination of prescription orthotic devices, with or without heel raises, may be required.

Major structural discrepancies—the legs differ in length by more than can be accommodated with shoe modifications—require dramatic limb-lengthening surgery. If you require this type of surgery, you will be referred to an orthopedic surgeon. Highly specialized centers perform limb-lengthening surgery. Briefly, the procedure involves cutting through the bones to be lengthened and inserting rods or surgical pins above and below the bone cut. These rods are slowly levered apart from each other to lengthen the bone by about 1 millimeter a day, which is slow enough to allow the nerves, muscles, tendons, and blood vessels to gradually elongate without injury.

Chapter 5

Flat Feet and
High-Arched Feet

TWO PROBLEMS WITH FOOT alignment are relatively common: having a foot with a low or no arch, usually described as a flat foot, or having a foot with a very high arch, also known as a pes cavus, or simply cavus, foot. Of the two, flat foot is the more common. The foot misalignment generally occurs on both sides, so that a person has either two flat feet or two cavus feet. The exception is with some neuromuscular conditions, such as cerebral palsy and stroke, where only one side may be affected. Each condition has its own set of causes, symptoms, and treatment options.

No Arch: A Flat Foot

When the arch of the foot lowers or completely collapses so that the entire sole of the foot contacts the ground, the condition is called flat foot, as shown in figure 5.1. Using the terms introduced in chapter 1 and also discussed in chapter 4, a flat foot is an overpronated foot. The ankle rolls inward while the heel bone angles outward into the position called hindfoot valgus. Because the inner edge of a flat foot is low to the ground, or even contacts the ground, the shoe wears down on the inside of the sole. From behind, an observer can often see the toes pointing outward, the "too many toes" sign. Some people

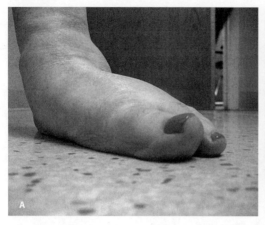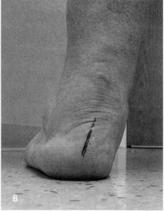

Figure 5.1. A flat foot is in an over-pronated position. Note the collapsed arch touching the ground in (A).

with flat feet are unable to rise up onto their toes, and upward movement of the foot at the ankle (dorsiflexion) may be restricted.

When walking, a flat foot fails to become the rigid lever needed for push-off. This limitation decreases the foot's ability to transfer weight to the front of the foot and diminishes the efficiency of forward motion. When a foot remains in a pronated position for a prolonged time, the lower leg rolls inward and creates a domino effect up the body with internal rotation of the knee, thigh, hip, and back. The repetitive rotational forces experienced by these parts of the body place additional strain on the muscles, tendons, and ligaments of the lower leg and foot.

People have or develop a flat foot for numerous reasons. They may have a foot type that leads to the condition. For example, they may have loose or weak ligaments encompassing the joints that connect the foot bones, or they may have abnormal connection between two bones that should be separate, a situation referred to as a *tarsal coalition*. They may have a tight or short-ened Achilles tendon (called ankle equinus), an injury that stretched or tore tendons and ligaments in the foot, or a past foot fracture. Muscle weakness from a nerve entrapment syndrome in the lower back, lower leg, or foot can also cause a flat foot. Additional causes are normal aging, arthritis, diabetes, obesity, neuromuscular conditions like stroke and cerebral palsy, pregnancy, or steroid use.

Symptoms of a flat foot range from mild to severe depending on the degree of deformity and how long you have had a flat foot. Children with a flat foot, and sometimes adults too, often complain about leg cramping, foot fatigue, or calf discomfort. Children may also refrain from participating in gym or recreational activities because of these symptoms. Other common complaints are the feeling of walking on the inside of the foot; bulging on the inside of the shoe; swelling; difficulty standing or walking on uneven ground, standing on the toes, and moving the foot around in circles; pain on the inside of the foot and ankle; and pain in the heels, knees, hips, and lower back.

If a flatfoot condition goes untreated, several long-term repercussions in addition to pain may cause significant problems. The tendons and ligaments in the foot can become progressively weaker and may tear, leading to disabling arthritis. Over a long period, the uneven stress and pressure on your foot's joints lead to pain, inflammation, cartilage damage, and loss of motion in the foot and ankle joints (see chapter 11). As the flatfoot condition progresses, your foot may even lose its flexibility and become rigid, which limits its ability to function as a shock absorber and adaptor to changes in the contour of a walking surface.

When assessing a flat foot, a podiatrist may use various diagnostic imaging techniques, such as x-ray, magnetic resonance imaging (MRI), and computerized tomography scan (CT scan), to identify contributing soft tissue or bone abnormalities. Diagnostic imaging also helps determine an appropriate surgical procedure to correct your flat foot if it has not responded to conservative, nonsurgical care.

Initial treatment for a flexible flat foot aims to restore or improve your foot's position and to relieve the pain and inflammation. The podiatrist may suggest that you wear shoes with greater arch support, use an over-the-counter or custom-made orthotic or brace, or take nonsteroidal anti-inflammatory medication. Many shoe companies design lines of motion control shoes, which are specifically made to address the needs of a flat foot. If these initial treatments aren't successful, especially if you have associated muscle weakness, arthritis, or tendon injury, then you may benefit from physical therapy. Physical therapy can help improve your foot's range of motion, balance, pain, and muscle strength. If yours is a nonresponsive case, the podiatrist may recommend bracing with an ankle–foot orthotic, such as a Richie brace, to provide additional support, offload pressure, and control the hindfoot. Ankle–foot orthotics are discussed in chapter 16.

Nonsurgical treatment for a longstanding flat foot that has become fixed and arthritic focuses on diminishing the pain and accommodating the foot so that you can remain as mobile as possible. Treatment can include nonsteroidal anti-inflammatory medication, cortisone injections into painful joints, orthotics, braces, physical therapy, or shoe change or modification. The actual position of a rigid flat foot can only be corrected with surgery.

Surgery is reserved for feet that do not improve with several months of conservative, nonsurgical care. Various surgical procedures are designed to reduce pain and improve the position and function of the foot. The procedure is customized on a case-by-case basis, depending on the extent and rigidity of the flat foot; the degree to which muscles, tendons, and ligaments contribute to the condition; and the presence or absence of arthritis in the joints. Typically, surgery for a flexible, nonarthritic flat foot involves lengthening a shortened Achilles tendon, making corrective bone cuts, and transferring tendons to support a weakened posterior tibial tendon. Surgery for a rigid, arthritic flat foot usually involves fusing bones that are normally separated by a joint. The recovery time is similar for both types of surgery, with ten to twelve weeks of immobilization and not putting any weight on the foot, and then a gradual return to protected weight bearing in a surgical walking cast. You must be prepared for full recovery to take at least six to twelve months after surgery.

Tendonitis Associated with Flat Feet

A longstanding flatfoot condition frequently results in a tendon injury called *posterior tibial tendonitis,* most commonly seen in middle-aged, overweight females, although it can occur in anyone with an excessively flattened foot. The posterior tibial tendon originates from a muscle in the inner portion of the leg below the knee. It runs behind and under the inner ankle to insert into the bones on the inside and under portion of the midfoot at the arch. The tendon resists eversion (the sole of the foot turning away from the body's midline), stabilizes the arch in weight-bearing activities, and assists the foot with push-off during the gait cycle.

When the tendon is strained excessively, the tendon sheath or the tendon itself becomes inflamed. The tendon may lose its normal linear, parallel fiber arrangement, and attempt to heal itself by forming scar tissue. The tendon can become partially torn (often along its length), thickened by scar tissue, and weak, but complete rupture is unusual. As the problem progresses, the ligaments and lining of joints on the inside of the foot can also stretch. The weakness in the tendon causes the leg to rotate inward toward the midline of the body, the heel to evert so that the sole turns outward from the midline, and the forefoot to abduct, or move away from the midline. People with posterior tibial tendonitis often complain that they're unable to walk for any considerable distance or length of time. They also experience the unnerving sensation of losing their balance while getting up from a seated position and while walking, especially on uneven terrain. In addition, they're unable to rise up onto their toes.

A podiatrist diagnoses the condition with a physical examination and may order an MRI to evaluate the extent of tendon injury. Treatment of posterior tibial tendonitis is much the same as treatment of a flat foot. Rest, ice, and elevation help to reduce swelling and pain, while custom-made orthotics, braces, and supportive shoes limit pronation and support the arch. If yours is a severe case that won't respond to other treatments, it may be necessary to immobilize the foot. Immobilization can vary from a CAM walker (a walking cast like a rigid boot) to a below-the-knee plaster or fiberglass cast with crutches, both typically used for four to six weeks. Often, an ankle brace is used for three to six months after the initial casting to provide increased stability and protection as the patient returns to normal activity and exercise. Depending on the severity of the condition, some people need to continue using a brace for longer, occasionally for their lifetime.

If nonsurgical treatment fails to provide pain relief or improved function, you may decide to pursue surgical correction. Surgery usually consists of repairing or augmenting the posterior tibial tendon and realigning the foot. Tendon augmentation involves transferring a tendon from elsewhere in the foot or using a synthetic tendon graft.

High Arch: A Cavus Foot

The opposite of a flat foot is a high-arched foot, also called a pes cavus, or cavus, foot. The arch of a cavus foot is extremely high as a result of an imbalance in the muscles that support the foot or a skeletal abnormality. The foot may be flexible or rigid. In a flexible cavus foot, the arch appears to be abnormally high when the person is seated and reduces when standing. In a rigid cavus foot, the arch height does not change between sitting and standing.

The cavus foot occurs most frequently as an inherited structural condition. It is often associated with a neuromuscular disorder, such as cerebral palsy, muscular dystrophy, stroke, spina bifida, or polio. Other causes of a cavus foot include burns, infection, trauma, and compartment syndrome (a condition that leads to nerve damage by cutting off the blood supply to the nerves within a closed space, or compartment, in the body).

Various other problems occur for a person with a pes cavus foot. He or she may develop hammertoes or claw toes along with metatarsalgia (see chapter 8). The downward position of the forefoot relative to the hindfoot causes the extensor tendons that bring the toes up to tighten. This tightness pulls the toes up and forces down the metatarsal bone behind the toe, causing excess pressure, with possible pain and skin thickening (callus) under the ball of the foot. The two small sesamoid bones just behind the big toe may become inflamed, a condition called sesamoiditis (see chapter 14). Calluses can also develop on top of the toes, on the heel, and on the outside of the foot. The downward position of the forefoot can increase stress on the joints at the apex of the high arch, in the midfoot, leading over time to osteoarthritis, a degenerative joint disease (see chapter 11). In addition, a person with a cavus foot may have tightness in the Achilles tendon and in the soft tissues (the plantar fascia) supporting the arch. This tightness can cause pain in the bottom or back of the heel along with plantar fasciitis, Haglund's deformity, or Achilles tendonitis (all of which are discussed in chapter 9).

As well as the downward position of the forefoot, the front of the foot may curve toward the center of the body, creating a convex outer edge and a concave inner edge, the position associated with a forefoot varus. This curving of the foot places excess weight on the outer edge of the foot, which can be seen as the soles of shoes are worn down on the outside. Nerve entrapment syndromes (see chapter 10) can also result from a cavus foot, and when the cavus foot is of neuromuscular origin, there can be associated neuromuscular symptoms such as muscle weakness, drop foot (the inability to lift the foot; see chapter 4), burning, tingling, and pain. A person with any of these signs or symptoms may be referred to a neurologist. (Signs are what a doctor documents; symptoms are what a patient experiences.)

Walking is more difficult with a high-arched foot. A cavus foot is less able to pronate adequately when the foot contacts the ground, and therefore the foot is a poor shock absorber. Poor shock absorption can cause discomfort extending from the lower back to the lower leg, ankle, and foot. Stress fractures within the foot and lower leg occur more frequently. Ankle sprains are also more common, because the heel of a cavus foot turns inward toward the center of the body, creating ankle instability. Even treading on a small object or walking on slightly uneven terrain can cause an ankle sprain. A person with a cavus foot is often described as having a measured gait, because of the extra caution taken at each step. An inverted heel may also create tension and stretch in the tendons on the outer portion of the foot and ankle, leading to tendon inflammation, thickening, tearing, or displacement. Over time, the ankle joint may become inverted, which alters pressure distribution within the joint and can lead to osteoarthritis.

Treatment of a pes cavus foot is designed to reduce pain and improve function. Nonsurgical options include various shoe modifications: cushioned shoes with extra depth to accommodate hammertoes, high-top shoes to increase ankle support, shoe wedges on the outer portion of the sole or heel to reduce weight on the outer part of the foot, and rocker soles to decrease pressure on the ball of the foot. As with the flatfoot condition, many shoe companies design lines of shoes to address the needs of a cavus foot, largely to provide more cushioning. If you have a cavus foot, you may find a custom-made orthotic or an over-the-counter or custom-made ankle brace to be beneficial. Calluses can be treated as described in chapter 6, and physical therapy can address muscle weakness and tightness of the Achilles tendon or plantar fascia ligament. Treatment for neuromuscular conditions are discussed in chapter 10.

If your pain and instability continue despite exhausting the conservative treatment options, you may need to consider surgery. Surgery for a pes cavus

foot targets all soft tissue and bone abnormalities contributing to the condition. The procedures include tendon transfers to augment tendons that are
derived from weakened muscles, Achilles tendon lengthening, ligament repair, bone cuts for realignment, and corrective bone fusions. Surgical bone
fusions are typically suggested in cases where the cavus condition becomes
progressively worse over time, such as for people with certain neuromuscular
diseases, and in cases with severe degenerative changes within the joints.

Chapter 6

Skin Conditions Affecting
the Foot

THOUGH MANY OF US don't think of it as such, the skin is an organ with numerous functions. It encases our internal structures—organs, bones, muscles, blood vessels—and acts as a barrier against infection and other environmental influences such as chemicals. It helps to protect the body from sunburns and physical injury. It regulates heat loss and heat gain to keep the body's internal temperature at a relatively constant 98.6 degrees Fahrenheit. The skin also minimizes fluid loss, thereby helping to guard against dehydration. As a sensory organ, the skin helps us relate to our environment by feeling touch, pain, heat, and cold. It is even involved in the manufacture of vitamin D when it's exposed to the sun. In short, the skin is an extraordinary piece of evolutionary engineering.

The skin varies in thickness and structure depending on the needs of different parts of the body. For example, the skin that covers the eyelids has a very different function from the skin on the palms of the hands and soles of the feet. The skin on the feet must be tough enough to endure the repetitive pressure from walking and running, yet remain flexible enough for the foot and ankle to move and bend. In this chapter, we first describe the anatomy of the skin and then discuss the common skin conditions that affect feet, as well as treatment options and prevention measures for those conditions.

Anatomy of the Skin

There are two types of skin: thick skin, which is found only on the palms of the hands and soles of the feet, and thin skin, which is found everywhere else on the body. Both types of skin consist of the *epidermis* and the *dermis*. Below the dermis is *subcutaneous tissue*.

Epidermis

The epidermis is the outermost surface of the skin and has five layers, of which only the bottom, or basal, layer is alive and grows new cells. This cell growth is supported by nutrients and oxygen transported in blood vessels from the dermis. The basal layer contains several types of cells, including *keratinocytes*, which produce the protein that makes up skin cells, and *melanocytes*, which are the pigment cells that give skin its color and protect skin cells from ultraviolet light. Over a few weeks, the cells grown in the basal layer move through the four upper layers of the epidermis. As the cells move toward the surface, they are no longer in contact with the blood supply, and therefore they die. Cell size becomes smaller and smaller, and the cells' water content decreases until, when the cells reach the surface, they are nothing more than dry scales of protein called *keratin*. These keratinized cells act as a barrier between the body and the environment.

Dermis

The dermis, directly below the epidermis, consists of the *papillary* and *reticular* layers. Within these layers are found all the skin's structures, such as sweat glands; hair follicles; sebaceous glands (oil glands); nerve endings that sense pressure, pain, and temperature; and blood and lymphatic vessels. There are also collagen fibers that give these structures support, and elastin fibers that give skin its flexibility. The tubes, or ducts, of many of the structures in the dermis pass through the epidermis to reach the surface.

The Fat in Our Feet

Thick pads of fat on the ball of the foot (below the metatarsal heads) and on the sole of the heel absorb and dissipate shock, provide cushioning, and protect the foot from pain. The subcutaneous tissue in these areas is well defined and is thicker than elsewhere in the body. From the inside, the tissue looks like a fibrous honeycomb with fat filling each space. The honeycomb-like structure prevents fat cells from squishing out the sides of the foot with every step.

As we age, these fat pads can become thinner, or atrophied, and they may even shift position. For example, the fat pad below the ball of the foot can shift forward to the base of the toes, resulting in increased pressure or pain below the metatarsal heads. Other people develop harmless yet painful lumps around the sides of the heels caused by some of the fat cells escaping their fibrous honeycomb compartments. These *piezogenic papules* (pressure-generated lumps) occur most often in obese individuals and in people with severely pronated feet because of the extra pressure on the inner side of the heel.

Subcutaneous Tissue

Subcutaneous tissue, which is composed of fat cells within a fibrous mesh, lies below the dermis and is not actually part of the skin itself. The subcutaneous tissue is responsible for storing fat as an energy reserve, acting as a cushion for the body, and insulating the body from cold temperatures.

Bubbles of Pain: Blisters

At one time or another, everyone has experienced a blister on the heel or toe or side of the foot. Most blisters form from rubbing or friction across the skin. To understand how friction causes a blister, rub one finger over the top of your opposite hand. Rub lightly enough that the skin doesn't move very much. If you continue this action for long enough, heat will develop and a blister will form. This skin rubbing is exactly what happens to your foot in a shoe that's too tight or too stiff or even too wide. Friction blisters have a raised bubble of skin, usually filled with a clear fluid. Sometimes blisters fill with blood, making them appear red, purple, or black. Blisters can also occur as a result of allergies, fungal or bacterial infections, and reactions to medication. These blisters tend to be numerous and cluster in a particular spot on the foot and are often surrounded by reddened skin. If you experience blisters of this sort, refrain from self-treatment and consult a dermatologist or podiatrist. Other causes of blisters include burns, frostbite, and trauma (fracture blisters).

The best strategy with blisters is to prevent them from occurring in the first place. Prevention begins with wearing properly fitting shoes that do not create excess pressure or friction on the foot (see chapter 3 for more details on choosing properly fitting shoes). Wearing seamless socks also removes a potential source of friction. Another option is to wear double-layer socks or two socks. Friction is created between the layers of sock instead of between the sock and your foot. Synthetic socks wick moisture away from the foot better than cotton socks do, which is important because moist skin is more susceptible to injury. If your feet sweat a lot, use an antiperspirant, cornstarch, or talcum powder on them. Cover areas that consistently blister with tape, silicon pads, or moleskin to prevent irritation. Lastly, petroleum jelly, A and D ointment, or an equivalent product can be used to decrease friction on the foot.

A friction blister filled with clear fluid can be treated safely at home in many cases (except for people with diabetes or poor circulation). First, wash your hands and the affected area of your foot with an antibacterial soap and water. Clean a needle with rubbing alcohol, betadine solution, or hydrogen peroxide, or hold the needle in a flame and then allow it to cool. Once the needle is clean, puncture the blister to allow the clear fluid to drain. Leave the blistered skin intact because it acts as a sterile dressing. If the blister continues to refill even after puncturing, remove a very small piece of the blistered skin while leaving the remaining skin flap intact. After draining the blister, clean the skin with antibacterial soap and water, apply a topical antibiotic such as triple antibiotic ointment, and cover the blister with a Band-Aid or gauze. While the blistered area heals, eliminate the activity or source of friction that caused the blister. If a blister is slow to heal, if you have poor circulation or diabetes, or if you note an increase in redness, pain, and swelling (signs of infection), then see a podiatrist. Blood within a blister is usually a sign of deeper skin damage. In this case, as well as when a blister forms as a result of infection, allergy, frostbite, or trauma, the safest option is to seek medical attention.

Thick Skinned: Corns and Calluses

Corns and calluses appear on the feet as a result of the skin becoming thickened, known as *hyperkeratosis*. *Hyper-* means excessive and *keratosis* refers to keratin, a protein that makes up hair and skin. Therefore, with hyperkeratosis there is an excessive accumulation of skin. In contrast to blisters that are caused by friction, the thickened skin of corns and calluses is caused by shearing. Shearing also can be demonstrated by rubbing one finger over the back of your opposite hand. This time, press firmly enough to move the skin and subcutaneous tissues; they are pinched between your finger and the bone below the skin on the back of the hand. This movement of the pinched skin is shear, which makes the skin adapt by growing more rapidly. In normal circumstances, skin cells move toward the surface, losing fluid and becoming flatter so that they effectively turn into scales of keratin, forming a protective layer that allows the skin to withstand such forces as friction and shear.

Since it is continuously being replaced, we can use the surface of the skin without the worry of wearing it out. However, if placed under a greater than normal load, the skin will grow more rapidly so that keratin builds up faster than it's sloughed off, and a corn or callus will form. At an acceptable level, this extra, or thickened, skin provides greater protection for the individual. For example, laborers and gymnasts, as well as barefoot dancers and tight-rope performers, who repetitively use the same surfaces of their hands or feet benefit from a protective callus to prevent painful blisters from forming. Too much buildup of extra skin, though, can lead to painful corns and calluses and even fissures (cracks) in the skin that can increase the risk of bacterial infection. Although both calluses and corns result from excessive skin building up at a place on the foot that's subject to repetitive shearing pressure, they differ in appearance, symptoms, and treatment.

Calluses

Calluses typically appear as areas of hard skin on the sole of the foot. They are spread out, or diffuse, covering a fairly large area, and the skin lines are usually enlarged or prominent, as seen in figure 6.1. A callus may not cause any symptoms, in which case you can ignore it unless you have diabetes, poor circulation, loss of protective sensation in the foot, neuropathy, or peripheral arterial disease. In other cases, however, a callus causes a dull, annoying, burning sensation. Calluses can be self-treated by filing the excess thickened skin with a pumice stone or emery board. You can use any of the numerous over-the-counter devices that resemble shavers, such as the Ped Egg, provided you are not in the risk group listed above. After filing the skin, moisturize the area with an over-the-counter emollient; products that contain lactic acid, urea, or lanolin are all very good softeners. Soft insoles can provide additional cushioning for a callus on the sole of the foot. Pads can also be added to over-the-counter insoles or to the shoe's regular insoles to take weight off a painful callus.

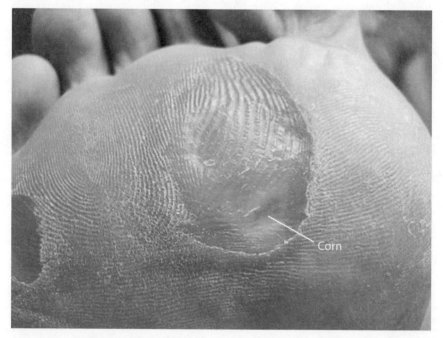

Figure 6.1. A callus has enlarged skin lines. This lesion has a corn within the callus.

Corns

Corns usually develop over a smaller area and are deeper than calluses. As with calluses, skin lines remain. When the thickened skin forms on top of or between the toes, it is commonly referred to as a hard corn, or *helloma dura*, shown in figure 6.2A. Hard corns usually form on top of prominent knuckles associated with hammertoes because of pressure from shoes. Hard corns between the toes are generally due to pressure from adjacent toes. When a corn forms deep within a web space between the toes, perspiration can soften it and cause a white and macerated appearance. These corns are referred to as soft corns, or *helloma molle*.

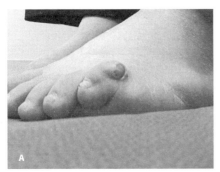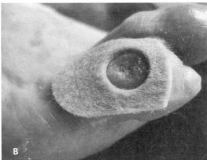

Figure 6.2. (A) A hard corn (helloma dura) on the fifth toe. (B) An aperture pad applied around a removed corn.

Both hard and soft corns can vary dramatically in the discomfort they cause; they can be painless, mildly tender, or acutely painful and burning. The severity of the symptoms is often related to the depth of the corn and whether a bursitis has developed below it. (A bursitis is the inflammation of a small sac, called a bursa, that lies between the skin and a bone or tendon.) A bursitis is usually present if the pain intensifies when the area below the corn is gently squeezed from side to side rather than when pressing on top of the corn.

Corns can be safely treated at home, except if you have diabetes, poor circulation, loss of protective sensation in the feet, or a compromised immune system. If you are in one of these situations, go to a podiatrist for relief from a painful corn. Self-treatment includes gentle filing with an emery board, which is best done after bathing, when the skin is softer. Never use sharp instruments on a corn. After filing, apply aperture pads around the edges (not directly on the corn) to relieve pressure on the area, as shown in figure 6.2B. Corn patches contain salicylic acid and can be applied to a hard corn (*not* to a soft corn). The acid softens and eats away at the corn, eventually allowing you to peel off the lesion. The patch must be cut to the exact size of the lesion so that normal skin is not damaged. Do not use these patches in the web spaces between the toes because the skin can become macerated and is then more likely to become infected. To reduce inflammation and pain, use ice and nonsteroidal anti-inflammatory medications, such as ibuprofen and naproxen. Last, avoid tight or poorly fitting shoes to minimize the chance of a corn recurring.

If symptoms fail to improve within several weeks of self-treatment, we recommend that you see a podiatrist for care. A podiatrist will most likely trim the hard skin with a scalpel, apply padding to the surrounding area, and possibly infiltrate the inflamed tissue below the corn with a weak cortisone solution to reduce inflammation, thereby shrinking the bursa and reducing the pain. Most often, the conservative treatments of filing, trimming, and padding are sufficient to treat a corn. However, if these measures fail, then surgery may be necessary. If the podiatrist suspects that an underlying bony prominence, such as a spur or hammertoe, is the cause of the corn, then an x-ray may be required to evaluate it. In these cases, simply trimming the corn is not a long-term solution because it will re-form within a matter of weeks. Therefore, the underlying cause needs to be addressed. Many of the conditions that cause corns (and calluses) to develop are covered in other chapters of this book, including bunions, hammertoes, and metatarsalgia (all in chapter 8) and flat foot (chapter 5).

Corn within a Callus

Occasionally, a callus will develop a thicker focal area, a so-called corn within a callus, as in figure 6.1. These lesions are typically exquisitely painful. When they form directly below a bony prominence, for example, below a metatarsal head, they are referred to as an *intractable plantar keratoma* (IPK). An IPK appears as a very deep, near-transparent lesion that leaves a depression in the foot when it's trimmed. These lesions are often confused with plantar warts, but warts have a cauliflower appearance and exhibit pinpoint bleeding after trimming. You should obtain professional care if symptoms fail to improve within several weeks of self-treatment, which includes filing, padding, and using cushioned insoles.

Another, less common kind of keratoma, a porokeratoma, will form adjacent to but not directly below a bony prominence. These lesions are also exquisitely painful. After trimming, they tend to have a moatlike white ring surrounding the corn as well as a near-transparent center. They are more likely to bleed than an IPK and are believed to be the result of a plugged sweat duct.

Conservative treatment for IPK and porokeratomas includes trimming and offloading the pressure with corn pads, modified over-the-counter insoles, or custom-made orthotics. Trimming typically provides relief for four to eight weeks, which can be prolonged to twelve weeks or more with the application of salicylic acid. Patches impregnated with salicylic acid are used in the same way as described above for hard corns. Curettage (surgically scooping out) of a porokeratoma is successful approximately 50 percent of the time, but curettage is not an option to treat IPK because the underlying cause is a bony prominence. If trimming, padding, and orthotic devices fail to provide adequate relief for an IPK, then you may need to consider surgical treatment. When a prominent metatarsal head is to blame, the surgical procedure elevates the head underlying the lesion.

Cauliflowers of the Skin: Warts

Warts are an extremely common reason for people to visit a podiatrist. They are classified as benign tumors of the epidermis and are caused by a virus (the human papillomavirus, or HPV). The virus invades the nucleus, or brain, of a cell and takes over its growth so that the skin begins to grow very rapidly. This rapid growth results in a buildup of keratin, which looks similar to a corn. However, a wart has a bumpy, cauliflower appearance, and on close inspection, you may be able to see small black flecks, which are dried blood clots from the capillaries. Unlike corns and calluses, warts obliterate normal skin lines.

It's sometimes necessary to trim a wart before you can distinguish it from a corn. As it's trimmed, the wart will exhibit pinpoint bleeding as the tiny capillaries caught between the exaggerated ridges of the epidermis are sheared off by the blade.

Warts often form in the same locations as corns and calluses, below weight-bearing bony prominences like the metatarsal heads. Yet, unlike corns and calluses, they may also occur in non-weight-bearing areas, such as below the arch and on top of the foot. Warts on the sole of the foot are called *plantar warts*, or in medical terms, *verruca plantaris*. Warts that occur on the top of the foot may be raised (*verruca vulgaris*) or flat (*verruca plana*). Warts can appear alone or in clumps of closely coalescing lesions referred to as *mosaic warts*. Mosaic warts are more likely to spread and are more challenging to treat. Warts may also appear as a large mother wart with multiple smaller satellites known as daughter warts. Typically, warts begin quite small and without symptoms, but as they enlarge, they frequently cause a sharp pinlike pain.

The HPV virus that causes warts is contagious, so it's possible to contract the virus and develop warts from walking barefoot in public showers, in locker rooms, and around pools, as well as in home showers shared with family members who have warts. Some people may be more prone than others to contracting an HPV infection. Once someone has had a wart, he or she seems to be more likely to have them in the future. People with immune system deficiencies are also more likely to contract warts. Some physicians think there may be a genetic link, but warts occurring on several family members may be simply the result of transmission through shared facilities.

Warts can be treated, but sometimes even aggressive treatment doesn't eliminate them. Self-treatment includes applying salicylic acid, which is available as a liquid film (similar to applying nail polish) and in patches. If you use the liquid, apply it daily and cover the area with a Band-Aid or tape. As the product accumulates, you can clip away the buildup, being careful not to cut the underlying skin. Continue until the wart has cleared up. If you use the patches, cut and apply them as described for corns. Patches are best applied after showering or bathing, when the skin is clean and hydrated, because the chemical penetrates the skin better. Treatment for plantar warts is basically the same as for other warts, except that the skin is thicker, and over-the-counter remedies are less likely to be successful. Children with plantar warts generally do well with a combination of home and professional care: The family applies the salicylic acid daily, and every second week the physician trims the lesion.

You should go for professional care if your warts persist, spread, bleed, become painful or infected, or fail to show signs of improvement within several weeks. A lesion that clears up and then recurs should also be evaluated by a physician. Some forms of skin cancer resemble warts so closely that even physicians can be fooled on initial treatment. Treatment by a podiatrist, family doctor, or dermatologist may include curettage and electrodesiccation (removing the wart with a small instrument that resembles a melon scoop and then electrically searing the area); cryosurgery, in which the wart is destroyed by freezing it, usually with liquid nitrogen; and chemical cautery, which involves applying or injecting strong chemicals.

Sometimes treating warts is like treating other tumors. Initially, chemicals may be used to shrink the growth, and when it is small enough, the remaining portion is cut out. Often a variety of remedies needs to be tried, and sometimes all forms of treatment are exhausted without success. Stubborn warts are biopsied to provide a definitive diagnosis. If you have a wart that continues to resist treatment or that recurs multiple times, a podiatrist may refer you for a second opinion and treatment by a different specialist, such as a dermatologist.

To minimize the chance of warts recurring, keep your feet clean and dry, powder your feet if they perspire heavily, and wear shoes in public places. Some physicians recommend cleaning home showers and even shoes with 10 percent bleach or Lysol and throwing out shoes if you have multiple recurrences, but there is no scientific evidence that these measures are effective.

Not Only for Athletes: Athlete's Foot

Athlete's foot, also referred to as *tinea pedis*, is another common skin problem that brings patients to a podiatrist. Essentially a ringworm of the feet, athlete's foot is an infection caused by fungi and yeast. There are thousands of strains of fungus, including the mushrooms you buy in the grocery store, yet only a few are pathogens (disease causing) in humans. The fungi responsible for athlete's foot are called *dermatophytes* and are present on our bodies in low numbers along with numerous types of bacteria. All of these fungi and bacteria are found within the uppermost layer of the epidermis.

Most of the time, the fungi on our skin don't cause any problems, but if we create an environment that favors their growth, then disease may develop. Fungi prefer warm, dark, moist environments, which happen to be the precise conditions found inside most closed shoes. The foot, therefore, is a frequent (but not the only) site of fungal infections. The risk of developing a fungal infection in the foot also increases with exposure to infested surfaces, such as public showers.

There are two forms of athlete's foot, an acute form that typically resolves quickly with self-treatment and a chronic form that is more difficult to eradicate and more likely to recur. The acute form is caused by a fungus with an impossibly long name: *Trichophyton mentagrophytes*. Infection by this organism typically manifests as tiny weeping blisters or slightly raised red bumps. This rash frequently occurs in the non-weight-bearing areas of the foot's arch, sometimes along the border of the foot, and less commonly on the top of the foot. The rash is usually very itchy (pruritic), and when it forms in the web spaces between the toes it can cause the skin to become macerated (mushy and white), to crack or fissure, and to have an offensive smell.

The chronic form of athlete's foot is caused by a related fungus, *Trichophyton rubrum*, and is often mistaken for dry skin. This type appears as a diffuse scaling and sometimes redness to the entire sole of the foot in a moccasin distribution. Chronic athlete's foot may not have any symptoms of pain or itching, but it can be a reservoir for the spread of infection to the toenails.

The acute form of athlete's foot generally responds well to self-treatment. The chronic form is often more difficult to treat and usually needs a longer course of care, typically requiring a podiatrist. Occasionally, treatment with an oral medication is required to eradicate a chronic infection. To treat either acute or chronic athlete's foot, you should wash your feet with soap and water and dry them thoroughly, paying particular attention to the web spaces. Once your feet are dry, apply an over-the-counter cream, such as Lotrimin (clotrimazole), Tinactin (tolnaftate), or Lamisil (terbinifine). Apply the cream twice daily, and the athlete's foot should resolve in one to four weeks. If the infection does not clear up within four weeks, visit a podiatrist for a prescription cream or oral medication. If the podiatrist prescribes an oral medication such as Lamisil capsules, the usual course of treatment is two weeks.

Once the infection is gone, it can be helpful, especially for people who perspire heavily, to apply an antifungal powder to the foot, between the toes, and inside the shoes every day to limit the chance of the infection recurring. You can minimize the chance of contracting athlete's foot by alternating the shoes you wear from day to day and by wearing shoes in public places. Some people perspire excessively, a condition known as *hyperhidrosis*, so the use of a topical lotion or solution containing aluminum chloride (which requires a prescription) will help them maintain drier feet and web spaces. If you are in this situation, change your socks two or three times a day, and wear synthetic socks, which wick away moisture better than cotton socks.

To Scratch Where It Itches: Dermatitis

Just about everyone knows the irritation of having badly itchy skin. Itchiness, known medically as *pruritus*, is an extremely common skin problem and is really a symptom of *dermatitis*, a general term that means "inflammation of the skin," or a skin rash. Dermatitis and the resulting itchiness occur due to a mild stimulation or irritation of the skin from a host of causes. Allergies to inhaled substances, such as plant pollens, animal dander, and airborne environmental contaminants frequently cause dermatitis. Insect bites also cause itchiness in many people, as can contact allergies to animals, metals, glues, dyes, and even detergents and soaps. Some people experience dermatitis and itchiness from foods they eat. Dry skin, eczema, and some fungal infections can also result in itchiness for some people, particularly older individuals and people with diabetes and other metabolic disorders.

People perceive the severity of an itch differently, and the individual response varies widely. Excessive scratching can lead to thickening and discoloration of the skin (*lichenification*), and for some people, usually those with a psychological disorder, can progress to a neurodermatitis resulting in bleeding and infection. A podiatrist or dermatologist can usually identify the cause of dermatitis and itchiness by taking a patient's medical history and by examining the skin. Sometimes, the physician needs to take a biopsy of the skin and subcutaneous tissue to make a diagnosis.

If dry skin is the problem, an over-the-counter topical cream or lotion containing urea, lactic acid, or glycerin can be helpful. If you have dry skin on the feet, or elsewhere, try showering or bathing every second day instead of every day, limiting the time you spend soaking in the bathtub, and using a moisturizing soap like Dove or Caress. Mild cases of dermatitis and itchiness, and those caught early on, can be self-treated with an over-the-counter 1 percent hydrocortisone cream, although you should be aware that cortisone may mask an infection and can even inhibit the body's ability to fight infection. We don't recommend self-treatment if you have diabetes, poor circulation, or a compromised immune system. If you do, or if over-the-counter remedies are not resolving your itchiness, visit a dermatologist or a podiatrist. A specialist will treat dermatitis and itchiness usually with topical cortisone creams, moisturizing creams, lotions, and shampoos, and occasionally with antihistamines or oral steroids.

Skin conditions that result in crusting and scaling fall into the category of *exfoliative dermatitis* and include psoriasis, eczema, contact dermatitis, and drug allergy. We recommend that anyone with one of these skin disorders consult a dermatologist.

Injuries from the Cold: Chilblains and Frostbite

Chilblains (*pernio*) and frostbite are thermal injuries caused by exposure of the skin to cold temperatures. Of the two, chilblains are more common and less serious, but both can result in tissue damage. The feet and hands are frequently the sites of these thermal injuries because of the body's response to the cold.

Chilblains

When exposed to the cold, the blood vessels that feed the skin on the hands and feet constrict (their diameter decreases). This constriction limits the amount of blood, and therefore heat, that goes to the extremities and is lost into the air. Starved of adequate blood flow, some of the skin cells die, and chilblains appear. The areas affected by chilblains usually appear purple or dark red in color. These areas will still blanch when touched, and the color will gradually return to the purple or deep red hue when pressure is released.

Initially, chilblains will be painful, and later, after several days or even weeks, they may become intensely itchy. In some cases the skin may blister, peel, or even ulcerate (become an open wound). Some people are more prone to developing chilblains than others, particularly those individuals with Raynaud phenomenon, which is an overactive response to the cold that results in profound constriction of blood vessels.

When chilblains occur, limit further exposure to the cold to avoid permanent tissue damage. Gently warm the affected body part by placing a warm (*not* hot) heating pad somewhere near it but not on it. For example, if your toes are affected, place the heat source behind the knee to dilate (open) the blood vessels to the foot. Also, keep your skin clean and protected from pressure, such as the pressure of tight socks, to limit damage. You can treat the pain, itchiness, and discomfort of chilblains with nonsteroidal anti-inflammatory medication and lotions containing aloe vera. A podiatrist or family doctor may treat chilblains by prescribing a vasodilator, which is an oral medication that releases the spasm, or constriction, in the blood vessels. For example, a nitroglycerin patch can be applied over the main blood vessel that feeds the damaged area. In the case of chilblains on the sole of the foot or toes, the patch would be placed over an artery that runs along the inside edge of the heel behind the anklebone.

To prevent chilblains, wear woolen socks and thermal or insulated boots for outdoor winter activities. Avoid nicotine, caffeinated beverages, and chocolate (which has an ingredient similar in effect to caffeine), all of which are potent blood vessel constrictors, for several hours prior to engaging in outdoor activities during the winter months. You might like to try a small heat pad that activates by ripping open the package. Some people find these pads helpful when placed inside a ski or skate boot. Use them with care, however, to avoid causing blisters or wounding the skin, and don't use them at all if you have diabetes, peripheral vascular disease, or peripheral neuropathy. If you have recurring chilblains, a podiatrist may order blood tests to investigate possible reasons, such as the presence of cryoglobulins, which are proteins formed in the blood after exposure to the cold. These proteins may damage blood vessels, leading to chilblains.

Frostbite

Frostbite is more serious than chilblains, because it results from actual freezing of the skin and soft tissues, such as subcutaneous tissue, nerves, blood vessels, and tendons. The fluid outside the cells freezes, causing fluid inside the cells to leak out. The cells then dehydrate and die. Damage to the blood vessels allows blood to leak into the surrounding tissue, creating inflammation, swelling, and increased tissue injury. In addition, clots can form within the blood vessels, further reducing the amount of oxygen that reaches the tissues. When a body part is frostbitten, it initially feels cold, and the skin appears pale and waxy. As the skin begins to thaw, the frostbitten area may be red and have tiny blisters (*vesicles*) or larger blisters (*bullae*). The area is also likely to be painful.

A frostbite injury may be superficial, which is less serious, or deep, which can lead to irreversible tissue death known as gangrene. If the skin is pink and has clear blisters and dimples, the frostbite is likely superficial. If the skin is waxy and dark, has blood-colored blisters, and is firm or nonyielding, the injury is more likely to be deep. It may take days, weeks, or even months to know the full extent of the damage. Regardless of how the skin looks, frostbite should be treated as an emergency and by trained medical professionals. Until medical care is available, transport the individual to a warm environment and remove wet or constrictive clothing and jewelry. Do not attempt to warm the frostbitten skin if there is any chance of refreezing, because the outcome can be dramatically worsened. Keep the affected body part elevated to reduce further swelling, and to avoid further tissue damage, refrain from rubbing or massaging the skin. Keep in mind that someone with frostbite may also be experiencing hypothermia, so try to hydrate the person with warm fluids such as soup. Avoid chocolate and caffeinated beverages because of their constricting effect on blood vessels. Over the years, there has been controversy about whether to warm a frostbitten area rapidly or slowly; the current advice is not to warm the area at all and immediately seek professional assessment.

On the Surface: Skin Spots, Growths, and Lesions

Each of us has numerous spots, growths, and lesions on our skin, but fortunately, few are ever cause for concern. Nevertheless, every year many people are diagnosed with skin cancers, some of which are deadly. Treatment success is directly related to how early a diagnosis is made, and self-examination is the single most important aspect in arriving at an early diagnosis. With knowledge about different spots and what to look for, most people can determine whether a skin lesion is of sufficient concern to seek medical advice.

Solar Keratosis

Solar keratosis, also called *actinic keratosis*, not surprisingly occurs from the effects of the sun. A keratosis is simply an overgrowth of skin tissue containing the protein keratin. Solar keratoses look like slightly raised, rough, red lesions and are usually covered with a white scale. They range in size from slightly smaller to slightly larger than a pencil eraser. Typically, solar keratoses are found on individuals with fair complexions who have a long history of sun exposure. They commonly occur on the top of the foot and front of the leg. A small percentage of these lesions may progress over a period of years to decades to a form of skin cancer known as *squamous cell carcinoma*. Treatment options include cryosurgery, which is freezing with liquid nitrogen to destroy the lesion; topical anticancer skin preparations that are prescribed and applied by a physician; curettage, which is surgically scraping out the lesion; and surgical excision, which involves removing the lesion and suturing the edges of skin to cover the area. If you suspect a solar keratosis on your foot or leg, make an appointment with a podiatrist or, better yet, a dermatologist.

Seborrheic Keratosis

Seborrheic keratosis refers to lesions that are raised, with a typically warty texture; light to dark brown or black in color; and often waxy. They resemble actinic keratoses, but they are not caused by the sun. Seborrheic keratoses tend to occur in families and are benign (noncancerous). They do not require treatment, unless they are irritated by clothing.

Pigmented Spots

The color of our skin, as well as the color of our eyes and hair, is determined by pigment cells called melanocytes. When dense clusters or nests of melanocytes occur in the skin, the result is a *nevus* (plural *nevi*). Commonly referred to as birthmarks or moles, nevi are most often benign lesions, although they can become malignant over time. Another type of spot, also formed by an increased number of melanocytes, though not a dense cluster as with a nevus, is called a *lentigo* (plural *lentigines*). A lentigo is a small, well-defined, flat brown to black spot. There are several types of lentigines, some benign, some potentially malignant. One benign type, which commonly occurs in older people, is often referred to as an age spot.

Dreaded Words: Skin Cancer

Whether on the skin of the foot or anywhere else on the body, skin cancer of any type needs to be identified swiftly for best treatment outcomes. A helpful guide, especially for identifying malignant melanoma or atypical nevi, is the "A–B–C–D–E" characteristics of nevi. A "yes" response to one or more of the following questions may indicate a problem. If you're concerned, make an appointment to see your family doctor, a podiatrist, or a dermatologist.

Asymmetry: If a line is drawn through the middle of the lesion, do the two halves look different?
Borders: Are the borders or margins of the lesion indistinct, scalloped, irregular, or notched?
Color: Does the lesion vary or change in color, including brown, tan, black, red, blue, or white?
Diameter: Is the lesion increasing in size? If the lesion is a nevus, has it increased in diameter to greater than 6 millimeters, or larger than a pencil eraser?
Elevation: Is the lesion raised above the skin?

Additional sources of concern include lesions that are enlarging or bleeding and sores that won't heal. A nevus or other spot should be removed and biopsied if it's located in an area irritated by clothing or footwear, in an area that's not easily monitored, or on the weight-bearing parts of the feet (heel, ball of the foot, bottom of the toes).

A world-renowned melanoma researcher and surgeon once said to one of us, "There is no such thing as 'watch it.' Watch what? Watch it turn into cancer? If it needs to be watched, it needs to be removed." Given the frequency of moles and growths on our bodies, many of us will require an evaluation at some time in our lives. We certainly don't want to be alarmist and have every growth removed, but it's prudent to be aware and attentive to lesions. If you're suspicious of a lesion, consult a medical professional.

Treatment of a malignant skin lesion depends on the type of cancer; the size, depth, and location of the lesion; and the stage of development. Certain types of skin cancer are less invasive and once biopsied require no further treatment other than periodic monitoring. Others may require staging, which means evaluating whether the cancer has spread to lymph nodes or other parts of the body. Tools used by physicians in this evaluation include sentinel node biopsies, positron-emission tomography (PET) scans, and other imaging studies. Once the staging process has been completed, an oncology consultation with a team of medical professionals results in an appropriate treatment protocol recommendation. The team may include a radiation oncologist, medical oncologist, surgical oncologist, and, depending on the location and the extent to which the foot is involved, a podiatrist.

Basal Cell Carcinoma

The most common skin cancer is *basal cell carcinoma*, believed to be primarily caused by episodic exposure to the sun. This carcinoma usually occurs on the face, but it can also affect the top of the foot. (It is particularly important to protect the top of your foot with sunscreen, because the skin in this area is exposed directly to the sun.) Fortunately, a basal cell carcinoma rarely spreads to other locations. The appearance can vary, but typically, the lesion begins as a small, semitransparent, raised, waxy or pearly nodule with a central depression or crater. The overlying skin may be coursed by tiny blood vessels, looking like spider veins and known medically as *telangiectasias*, and the borders typically appear rolled. As the lesion grows, a crust may form over the central depression, and if the crust is pulled loose, the lesion bleeds.

Treatment options depend on the size and location of the lesion. It may simply require surgical excision and, if the lesion was large, skin grafting to cover the excised area. Curettage, or scooping out the lesion with a tool that electrically burns the base, is an option that provides a tissue specimen for biopsy and allows the wound to heal slowly without stitches. Other options, neither of which provide a tissue specimen for biopsy, are cryosurgery, or freezing, of the lesion or application of topical chemotherapeutic agents. The chemotherapeutic is incorporated by the rapidly growing tumor cells, and it poisons and kills them.

Squamous Cell Carcinoma

Squamous cell carcinoma is a skin cancer with more significant ramifications than basal cell carcinoma. A squamous cell carcinoma resembles a wart, with its cauliflower appearance, and is often slightly red in color, raised, and scaly, as in figure 6.3. These carcinomas tend to occur on sun-exposed skin and often begin as a solar keratosis that becomes malignant. Some forms of squamous

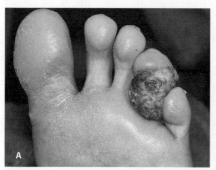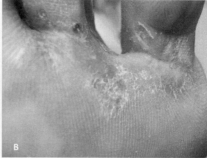

Figure 6.3. (A) A squamous cell carcinoma can resemble a wart. The lesion in this photo rapidly increased in size and bled, indicating a condition more serious than a wart. (B) This squamous cell carcinoma was diagnosed with a biopsy after topical antifungal medications did not clear up the lesion.

cell carcinoma don't spread and are referred to as an *in situ* carcinoma, or Bowen disease. This form requires only local treatment to cut the carcinoma out. Other squamous cell carcinomas are more serious. As a lesion grows in size over several months, it may begin to ulcerate and bleed. Like many malignant lesions, a squamous cell carcinoma is movable initially—meaning that it can be moved back and forth when gently touched—but as it invades the tissue below, it becomes more anchored and immovable. As the carcinoma spreads, it can invade the subcutaneous tissue, tendons, and bones. It may also spread to lymph nodes and internal organs if the lesion remains undiagnosed or if treatment is delayed. A squamous cell carcinoma is biopsied to determine how much tissue is involved, and depending on the location, the carcinoma may be removed with wide margins ("margins" in this context means tissues that contain no cancer cells). If there isn't enough tissue to close up the area after removing the lesion, it may be necessary to amputate a toe or part of the foot.

Malignant Melanoma

Malignant melanoma is the most serious of all skin cancers because of its propensity to spread. The cancer begins in the pigment cells, or melanocytes, that cluster to form a nevus, commonly known as a mole or beauty mark. Be suspicious when a mole begins to bleed, enlarge, elevate, or change shape or color. The color can vary among black, brown, red, white, and blue.

Malignant melanoma on the foot is more likely to occur in dark-skinned than in fair-skinned individuals. (Fair-skinned women tend to develop this melanoma on the lower legs, and fair-skinned men on the trunk.) When the melanoma occurs on the foot, it tends to be on the soles of the feet or below the toenails. A suspicious lesion under a toenail could be a benign pigmentation of the nail or of the skin below the nail, or it could be a *subungual hematoma*, which is blood trapped below the nail. A subungual hematoma can occur from a trauma, such as the nail rubbing against a shoe, and will grow out with the nail, eventually clearing up. A melanoma, as in figure 6.4, will not move with the growing nail. Diagnosis of a melanoma under a toenail may require a biopsy, which can permanently disfigure the nail. Once a malignant melanoma is confirmed, treatment options range from cutting out the melanoma with wide margins to amputation, depending on the depth of the lesion.

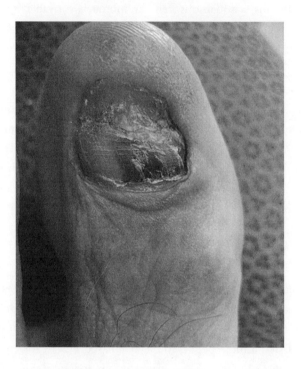

Figure 6.4. Trimming this toenail found no evidence of dried blood (subungual hematoma), and a subsequent biopsy confirmed malignant melanoma.

Chapter 7

Toenail Disorders

OUR TOENAILS ARE A vestigial structure, left over from our ancestors, who used them to hold onto objects or climb trees. They no longer are of significant use to us. Toenails do offer a measure of protection for the ends and tops of the toes, but shoes offer our toes far greater protection than even the healthiest toenails. Few people pay much attention to their toenails, beyond clipping them every so often—that is, unless their toenails become discolored, deformed, painful, or difficult to care for. As we age, many of us develop toenail problems, and basic toenail care can become more difficult. Thickened or very curved nails are hard to clip, and other issues like changing eyesight or arthritis in the hands can make nail clipping an awkward and frustrating task. Nevertheless, good nail care is essential for toenail health at any age.

This care includes proper trimming techniques, as well as wearing shoes and socks that fit well. Doing these simple things will go a long way toward keeping your toenails healthy, yet, despite your efforts, you still may develop a toenail disorder, perhaps because you sustain an injury or have a hereditary predisposition for such a problem.

In this chapter, we begin with a brief anatomy of the toenail so that you will recognize all its different parts as we describe the most common toenail problems, how to treat them, and how to prevent their recurrence.

Anatomy of a Toenail

A toenail (and fingernail) has three parts: the body, the root, and the free edge, or tip, all shown in figure 7.1. The *body of the nail* makes up most of what we see. It is attached to the skin underneath, which is termed the *nail bed.* Along each side of the nail body is the *border of the nail*, which rests in a *nail groove.* The skin alongside the nail border is termed the *nail lip.* The *root*, or *matrix*, of the nail is the only living portion. It begins next to the cuticle area and extends below the skin, going horizontally toward the foot. The leading edge of the root can be seen at the base of the nail as a small white crescent, or half moon. The root produces the new cells that become the body of the nail. The *free edge*, or *tip*, of the nail is the part that grows out at the end of the toe and gets clipped.

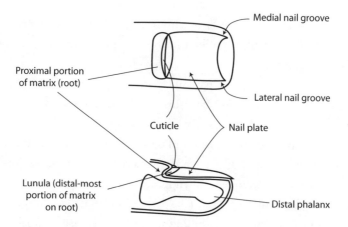

Figure 7.1. The parts of a toenail.

The entire nail, including the root, body, and tip, is often referred to as the *nail plate.* The skin below the nail tip is called the *hyponychium.* The cuticle area is the *eponychium.* The cuticle forms a seal between the nail and the skin and acts like a biological caulking material, preventing bacteria from invading the tissue around the nail, while still allowing the nail to grow.

Piercing the Skin: Ingrown Nails

Ingrown toenails are one of the most common reasons people visit a podiatrist. The condition occurs when the borders of the nail turn downward excessively and create pressure against the base of the nail groove. This pressure leads to the buildup of a callus between the nail border and the nail groove, causing inflammation, redness, swelling, and pain. An ingrown toenail affects the big toe most often, but it can happen to any toe. Figure 7.2 illustrates three toenails: a normal nail; an excessively curved nail, called a *crowned nail*, that has formed calluses in the nail grooves; and an ingrown nail that has penetrated the skin in one nail groove and will likely develop an infection.

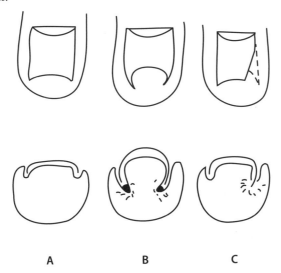

A   B   C

Figure 7.2. Toenails as seen from above and in front of the toe. (A) A normal nail plate with a flat body and minimally curved borders. (B) A crowned nail plate, where the borders create pressure at the base of the nail groove, resulting in a painful callus. (C) An ingrown nail, where one nail border has perforated the base of the nail groove.

Ingrown toenails develop for several reasons, including hereditary factors that affect the shape of the nail, trauma to the toes from stub injuries or dropped objects, and poor trimming technique. Trimming the nail too short or rounding the corners of the nail edge allows the skin to lift above the nail border and impede the forward growth of the nail plate. Although we recommend that you not round your toenails when trimming them at home, podiatrists commonly round the nails to relieve pressure and allow a patient to go longer between visits. Podiatrists use special instruments to round nails safely by leaving a smooth edge.

Repetitive pressure on the tips or sides of the toe can also cause ingrown toenails. For example, hammertoes and bunions (see chapter 8) can cause pressure to be applied to the nail plate from an adjacent toe, the shoe, or in the case of claw toes and mallet toes, the ground. Children and teenagers tend to have soft nails and often get into trouble by tearing instead of trimming their nails. When a toenail is torn by hand, the final piece of nail rips irregularly, resulting in a hook or sharp spicule of nail that pierces the skin as the nail grows forward (see figure 7.2C).

Self-treatment of a suspected ingrown toenail should be done with the utmost care—and *never* using sharp instruments—to avoid making the situation worse. If you notice any signs of infection—redness, odor, streaking, swelling, increased pain, or bleeding—then abandon self-treatment and see a podiatrist. If you are at increased risk of infection because of a compromised immune system, diabetes, or poor circulation, don't attempt to treat an ingrown toenail yourself. Instead, visit a podiatrist for care.

Self-treatment, including warm water soaks and topical antibiotic ointments, should relieve the pain within two or three days. Avoid wearing shoes and socks that place pressure on the nail border. Another safe and effective approach for treating an ingrown nail, especially with a crowned nail or an ingrown nail where the penetration is close to the tip of the toe, is one that we refer to as *nail lip taping*. After cleansing the area with soap and water and drying it well, place a piece of first-aid tape or the edge of a Band-Aid against the nail lip where it contacts the nail border. Draw the tape down and away to gently pull the nail lip away from the nail border, as in figure 7.3. The tape should relieve the pressure of the nail border against the inflamed nail groove, and within a day or so, the pain should be gone as well. Apply a small amount of topical antibiotic ointment in the nail groove, and place a second Band-Aid over the area to secure it. The ointment softens the callus in the base of the groove and reduces the chance of bacterial infection. The nail lip taping can be done until the pain subsides, usually within three to five days. We recommend that you seek care from a podiatrist if the pain, redness, swelling, and pus do not subside after three to five days of treatment at home.

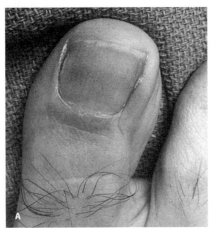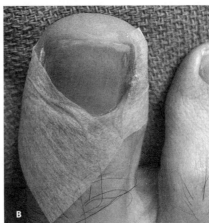

Figure 7.3. (A) Ingrown nail borders can be painful because of the callus that builds up in the nail groove. (B) Taping the nail lip away from the nail border for several days is usually enough to obtain relief.

Some of the old-time remedies are now frowned upon. One remedy was to place a wad of cotton under the edge of the nail to relieve pressure. Although this may give some relief initially, the cotton may harbor bacteria and increase the risk of infection. Cutting a V in the center of the nail plate has been advocated in the past, yet this too is ineffective. To relieve pressure at the nail borders, the V would have to extend to the cuticle area.

Once a toenail has penetrated below the surface of the skin, the body treats the nail as a foreign object and initiates its protective systems, sending white blood cells to the site to engulf and destroy the bacteria causing infection. The white blood cells consume microscopic foreign material and cell debris, creating pus, while other cells begin building a network of capillaries (minute blood vessels) around the area. The resulting bulge of tissue is called a *granuloma* and is commonly referred to as "proud flesh." A granuloma bleeds easily when pressure is applied to it, and it distorts the shape of the nail border. Sometimes, it can be painful. Eventually skin may grow over the granuloma, resulting in an enlarged nail lip. Once a granuloma forms, it is nearly impossible for a nail to grow out normally without surgical intervention.

Treatment for a granuloma requires professional care. A podiatrist will remove the ingrown portion of the nail (or other foreign object, if something else becomes embedded in the toe), usually with a local anesthetic in the physician's office. Once the nail or nail border has been removed, the podiatrist may take a swab of the area to culture the bacteria. The granuloma is then surgically cut out, or excised. Sometimes, a solution such as silver nitrate is also applied to shrink the tissue. In advanced cases, the granuloma and enlarged nail lip are cut away at the same time as the ingrown nail, while attempting to re-form the nail groove.

If you have an ingrown toenail treated in a podiatrist's office as described here, you can expect to walk out of the office after having the surgical procedure. The toe may stay numb for anywhere from three to eight hours, depending on the type of local anesthetic that was used. After surgery to remove an ingrown toenail, care for the toe and nail by soaking them twice daily in warm water (either fresh or salted), using dressings, and applying antibiotic creams or ointments to the affected area. The podiatrist will prescribe a course of oral antibiotics if infection spreads or if your immune system is compromised. Rarely do infections from an ingrown toenail require hospitalization, but occasionally, a delay in treatment can result in the spread of infection to bone. An otherwise healthy person probably doesn't require follow-up after surgery for an ingrown toenail, unless signs and symptoms of pain, redness, and pus fail to resolve within several days. If the infection had spread or you are at risk of infection, the podiatrist may ask you to return one or two weeks later to check the treated area. If a toenail continually becomes ingrown, the nail can be permanently partially or totally removed. Either the affected nail borders are permanently removed using chemical cauterization of the nail root, or the nail matrix is cut out.

Infection around the Nails

A bacterial infection that develops around a nail is referred to as a *paronychia*. Such infections can involve the entire cuticle area or one or both nail borders, as happens when an ingrown nail results in infection. A person with a paronychia complains of pain and redness. Sometimes the infected area oozes a small amount of pus, but other times pus is not present in the early stages of infection. In some cases, the nail is loose and discolored, but in others it looks normal. The infection can be the result of trauma to the toe or of an ingrown nail.

With the popularity of pedicures has come an increased incidence of toenail infection in young, healthy women. This increase may be due in part to the technique of pushing back cuticles. Because the cuticle forms a protective seal between the relatively hard nail plate and the soft skin and matrix surrounding the base of the nail preventing moisture and bacteria from getting below the skin, disturbing this protective barrier may allow infectious organisms to invade. Infection can also be transmitted through contaminated instruments. Some women purchase their own instruments to bring to salons when they receive a pedicure, but even these should be properly sterilized to minimize the risk of infection.

A paronychia is treated with warm compresses or soaks and antibiotic ointment. If it's associated with an ingrown toenail, the ingrown toenail needs to be treated as described above. Antibiotic ointment usually clears up the infection, but the portion of nail that loosened will not reattach, nor will the color be restored. However, as the new nail regrows, it will be attached and the color will return to normal, as long as the nail bed and nail matrix were not damaged.

Split in Two: Bifid Nails

When a nail splits along the length of the nail plate, it is referred to as a *bifid* nail. Bifid nails occur most commonly on the fifth toe and are believed to be caused by repetitive injury as the outside border of the nail rubs against the sole or side of the shoe during walking. This rubbing damages the root of the nail and causes it to grow in two pieces. Less often, bifid nails can be due to congenital influences or hereditary factors. Regardless of the cause, if the toe is rotated and the split nail continues to rub, a corn may develop below or adjacent to the nail. (See chapter 5 for information about corns.) Self-treatment of a split toenail includes trimming the nail or corn and using pads to protect the nail or corn from rubbing and to relieve pain from the rubbing pressure. If the pain is severe, a podiatrist can remove the abnormal nail, with or without a portion of the underlying bone, to reduce the pressure.

Blood under the Nail: Tennis (or Runner's) Toe

A fairly common trauma involves pressure on toes or repetitive bumping of toes inside a shoe, causing a subungual hematoma (blood under the nail), often called tennis toe or runner's toe. The blood under the nail makes the toenail look black, blue, brown, or dark red. Typically, subungual hematomas are not painful when they develop slowly from the repetitive micro-trauma of a toe bumping on a shoe. However, a subungual hematoma can also result rapidly from a macro-trauma, such as dropping something heavy on the toe; these injuries are extremely painful. Relief can be obtained by drilling holes—with or without a local anesthetic—to drain the blood away, but this procedure must be done soon after the injury, before the blood coagulates. If treatment is delayed, the nail is left to grow out, which could take many months, and may result in the nail plate separating from the nail bed. Sometimes, the whole nail sloughs off and a new nail grows. When a subungual hematoma (which occurs from a traumatic event) involves more than 25 percent of the nail bed, the nail should be removed to determine if the bed was torn or cut. If it was, it can be repaired with absorbable sutures.

Bones beneath the Nail: Spurs and Tumors

A painful condition can occur along the nail borders and under the tip of the nail when bony growths push upward from below the toenail. The most commonly affected digit is the big toe. Two types of abnormal bone growth can occur: a bone spur, called an *exostosis*, and a bone or cartilage tumor. *Subungual* means "under the nail," so a *subungual exostosis* is a bone spur beneath a nail. A bone and cartilage tumor under a toenail is called an *osteochondroma*. These tumors are benign (noncancerous).

A person with a subungual exostosis will have a painful circular area of red, brown, or pale yellow below the body of the nail closest to the tip. The toe is painful when wearing shoes and even from the pressure of bed covers, and the pain can also be felt when pressing a finger on the top of the toe. The pain is due to a corn that develops underneath the nail. A subungual exostosis can be misdiagnosed as an ingrown toenail or a toenail deformity, so a podiatrist may confirm the diagnosis by taking a special isolation x-ray. The podiatrist may also consider other conditions, such as warts and melanoma, that can mimic the signs and symptoms of subungual exostosis. Treatment of a subungual exostosis ranges from simply keeping the nail trimmed short and avoiding constrictive footgear to surgically filing or rasping the spur. This surgical procedure is usually performed in a podiatrist's office under local anesthetic. It is generally a permanent solution; recurrence of a subungual exostosis is rare. Recovery from the surgery is rapid; if you undergo surgical treatment of a subungual exostosis, you can generally expect to return to work, wearing an open sandal or surgical shoe, after a few days.

As with a bone spur, an osteochondroma typically arises from the bone below the nail plate, as shown in figure 7.4. This benign tumor of the bone or cartilage often mimics an enlarged nail lip, because the tumor on the bone pushes the skin up to the side of the nail groove. However, the area is very hard to the touch in comparison to an enlarged nail lip, which tends to be merely firm. Occasionally, a tumor grows large enough to perforate the skin. X-rays are used to confirm the diagnosis of an osteochondroma, and treatment requires surgical excision to remove the growth and reduce the chance of the overlying skin becoming damaged, because this can lead to a bone

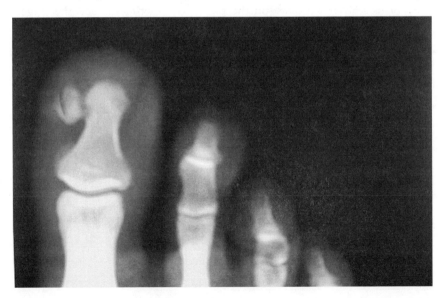

Figure 7.4. An x-ray showing an osteochondroma, a benign tumor of the bone or cartilage.

infection. This surgery requires more aggressive bone removal than surgery for a subungual exostosis, but the recovery time is similar. Recurrence of the problem is also rare.

Thick or Thin: Nail Dystrophy

Nail dystrophy refers to nails that become deformed, thickened, or thinned for a variety of reasons, including aging, trauma to the toes, and certain skin conditions. A person's blood circulation changes with age and causes nails to grow more slowly, resulting in a thickening of the nail plate. This thickening is entirely normal and doesn't require any treatment, unless the nail grows at an angle and cuts into the skin of adjacent toes, causes pain or a callus in the nail groove, or becomes so thick that it irritates or inflames the skin below the nail plate. You may simply find that your nails become more difficult to trim as they thicken, so you might consider going to a salon, unless you have a compromised immune system, diabetes, or poor circulation, in which case you should avoid salons.

Common skin conditions that may cause deformity to the nails include psoriasis and *lichen planus*. Psoriasis is a chronic, noninfectious skin condition that forms scaly red patches on the skin and sometimes affects the finger-nails and toenails, making them appear pitted or dimpled. When people with psoriasis have psoriatic nails, they often go on to develop psoriatic arthritis. Psoriatic nails tend not to require treatment, unless they become very thick or irregular and cause pain, in which case they can be thinned by electric grinding or removed. Inflammation or bacterial infection sometimes occurs because the irregular borders of the nail penetrate the nail grooves or the thickness of the nail elevates the cuticle.

Lichen planus is a noninfectious skin condition that forms a rash resembling a lichen (hence the name) on the skin and inside the mouth. The effects on the toenails can vary. In some cases, the nail matrix is damaged, and the nail thins, splits, and gets longitudinal ridges or grooves. In other cases, the nail can become severely thickened. If treatment is needed, it is the same treatment as for psoriatic nails.

Nail Fungus

Fungal infections of the toenails, called *onychomycosis*, are relatively common, affecting nearly one-fifth (18 percent) of people between ages 40 and 59, one-third (33 percent) between ages 60 and 70, and half (49 percent) over age 70. Given enough time and the right conditions, which include moisture, darkness, warmth, and repetitive injury to the nail plate, fungi that are found naturally in low numbers on the skin and around the nails can cause nail infection and deformity. The fungal spores can grow on top of the nail, below it from the nail tip, and within the matrix and nail bed. The organisms that cause fungal infections in nails are known as dermatophytes and may be the same ones that cause athlete's foot (see chapter 6). However, unlike athlete's foot, which develops rapidly after the skin is exposed to the responsible fungus, fungal infections of nails develop only after prolonged contact with the fungus. The people most prone to developing fungal nail infections are the elderly and individuals with a compromised immune system, including people with diabetes. Children are rarely affected.

Fungal infections of toenails can cause pain under the nail and at the borders if the nail becomes crowned, difficulty walking due to pressure on the nail from shoes, deformity and discoloration of the nail, and sometimes secondary bacterial infection. The unsightly appearance is often an issue as well, particularly for women who like to wear open-toe shoes. If left untreated, the fungal infection may spread to other nails.

There are three common types of onychomycosis. *Superficial white scaling onychomycosis* is an early form, which appears as a white scale on the surface of the nails. This infection is often first identified after removing nail polish that has been on the toenails for several weeks to months. The polish creates a wonderful breeding ground for fungus because it keeps out the light while locking in body heat, perspiration, and the moisture from showers or baths. Superficial white scaling may respond to topical treatment with antifungal creams or lotions, but they need to be used for a minimum of six to twelve months. Treatment should include scraping or filing away the scales or brittle bits of nail, twice daily cleansing, discontinuing the use of nail polish, and applying an over-the-counter or prescription topical antifungal cream (as described for athlete's foot). You might also find it beneficial to use a prescription lacquer, which is like a nail polish containing an antifungal agent. It may take weeks to months for the white scaling to grow out. To minimize the chance of recurrence, wash socks and treat shoes with antifungal powder. We also advise alternating pairs of shoes to allow perspiration to evaporate and the powder to work.

The second common type of fungal toenail infection is *distal subungual onychomycosis*. This infection is characterized by thickening or discoloration of the nail beginning at the tip or borders (the distal portions of the nail) but not extending to the half moon at the base. The infection spreads underneath the nail. This fungal infection is more difficult to eradicate with topical care than the superficial white scaling, but it is worthwhile to aggressively trim away all the affected nail and then try the same treatment described above. If that doesn't work, the entire nail can be removed. The nail bed is allowed to heal and then a topical antifungal cream is applied to the nail bed and nail plate as the nail regrows. Removing the nail takes away the barrier to the underlying nail bed, where the fungus grows, allowing the topical medications to work more effectively. Treatment is continued until the nail has completely regrown.

The third type of fungal infection, called *proximal subungual onychomycosis*, involves the entire nail. The infection begins at the base, or root (the proximal portion of the nail) and extends toward the sides and tip. The nail becomes very thick, and there is debris below the nail plate that may be yellow, white, brown, or black. Of the three types of fungal infection, proximal subungual onychomycosis is the most difficult to eradicate and usually requires an oral antifungal medication. However, before prescribing treatment with an oral medication, the podiatrist confirms the diagnosis by using a special staining technique, analyzing the nail microscopically, or culturing the fungus (which may take up to seven weeks to grow in an incubator). Once a proximal subungual onychomycosis is confirmed, you must undergo additional tests to assess your baseline liver and kidney function, because the medications used to treat this infection must be broken down by these organs, which in turn must be healthy for a person to take the medications safely. In addition, your medical and pharmaceutical history must be assessed to rule out contraindications with other health conditions or medications.

The treatment with oral medication continues for three months; laboratory tests are usually repeated midway through the treatment. The most commonly prescribed antifungal medications are terbinafine and itraconazole. We believe that of the two, terbinafine is superior in both effectiveness and safety. Both medications work by incorporating into the newly growing nail cells, thereby protecting them from becoming infected by the fungus. The appearance of the toenail won't improve until the old nail grows out, which occurs simultaneously with the new healthy nail growing in. The first signs of improvement may take up to three or four months to appear and will be visible at the root of the nail. The process of entirely replacing an infected toenail with a new, healthy nail can take as long as nine to twelve months. It's sometimes necessary to have an additional course of treatment for one to three months. In addition, it's important to note that the results can vary. Of people who use oral terbinafine, 40 to 90 percent can expect a mycological cure, meaning that the fungus is killed but the toenail continues to be thickened or doesn't look normal, and 35 to 50 percent of people have a clinical cure, which both kills the fungus and results in a normal-looking nail.

Once the affected nails are clear of fungus, keep a nail brush in the shower and gently scrub the toenails daily to keep the fungal count down. Alternating shoes from day to day, along with the periodic application of over-the-counter antifungal creams and powders, may also reduce the chance of a fungal infection recurring.

Chapter 8

Bunions and Other Toe Conditions

TOES CHANGE WITH AGE. As an adult, nobody expects to have the cute little toes of a baby, but neither do most people expect to develop one of the several toe conditions that tend to appear with age. Bunions and hammertoes are the two most common toe conditions, and both can be painful and disfiguring. Both conditions are inherited, and they generally become worse with age. Shoes themselves don't cause bunions or hammertoes to form, although they may contribute to their progression. In this chapter, we describe the causes, symptoms, and treatment options for bunions and hammertoes, as well as two forefoot conditions, metatarsalgia and predislocation syndrome.

A Bump on the Foot: Bunion

A *bunion* is a bump on the foot at the base of either the big toe or the little toe. A bunion at the base of the big toe is the *classic bunion* that most people think of, shown in figure 8.1A, and is the more common of the two types. A bunion at the base of the little toe is called a *tailor's bunion*, shown in figure 8.1B, so called because tailors of old sat cross-legged on the floor and frequently developed this problem from the constant pressure on the outer edge of their feet. You may also hear a tailor's bunion referred to as a bunionette.

Bunions are structural deformities where the framework of the foot is altered over many years.

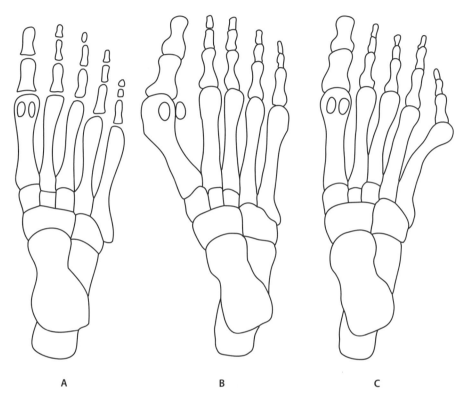

A   B   C

Figure 8.1. (A) A normal foot. (B) A classic bunion develops at the big toe joint. (C) A tailor's bunion develops at the base of the fifth toe.

Classic Bunion

A classic bunion develops from changes in the soft tissue and bone alignment within the joint where the big toe meets the foot, known as the first metatarsophalangeal joint. The metatarsal bones in the forefoot splay out, and the bone leading to the big toe, the first metatarsal, protrudes from inside the forefoot. As a bunion develops, the first metatarsal moves physically away from the adjacent bones, and excess bone accumulates at the site. The big toe slowly turns outward, angling away from the center of the body, and it encroaches on the adjacent toe. The soft tissues on the inside of the big toe joint, as well as the overlying skin, become stretched, while the soft tissues between the big toe and second toe become contracted.

A variation on the classic bunion is the *dorsal bunion*, which occurs when the bony prominence is located on top of the foot. In this case, the first metatarsal moves upward rather than inward. A dorsal bunion restricts the big toe's range of motion as the person walks, particularly at the toe-off phase of the gait cycle (see chapter 1). At toe off, the big toe jams against the first metatarsal at the big toe joint, instead of extending up and over the elevated first metatarsal as it normally should. Because of the limited motion by the toe, this condition is sometimes also termed *hallux limitus* or *hallux rigidus*. The causes, symptoms, and treatment options for a dorsal bunion are largely the same as for a classic bunion.

Numerous factors contribute to the development of a bunion, the main one being the type of foot a person has inherited. Certain foot structures are more prone to instability at the big toe joint, causing a bunion to develop gradually over the course of many years. Bunions are most commonly seen in people with flat feet and in people with excessive joint flexibility, termed a *hypermobile foot*. Other factors that contribute to the progression of bunions include tight or poorly fitting shoes; disorders of the nerves that control the muscles of the foot and ankle; trauma to the foot; inflammatory arthritis; and other disorders that affect connective tissues, such as the tendons, joint capsule, and ligaments around a joint. Tight or pointed shoes alone do not cause bunions. These types of shoes keep the big toe in an abnormal position, and they will irritate the skin and soft tissues over the bunion, or bump, causing pain. We know that shoes don't cause bunions because, although less common, people who have never worn shoes and those living where tight-fitting, western-style shoes aren't worn do develop bunions.

Bunions aren't always painful. Some people with bunions are free of symptoms. They may be concerned with the abnormal bone development only for cosmetic reasons. For other people, the main issue, again cosmetic, is the thickened skin (callus) underneath the prominent bone formation. However, for many individuals, bunions can cause significant symptoms that limit the activities they're able to enjoy. Symptoms may include pain, swelling, redness, burning, tingling in the big toe, loss of motion of the big toe, and pain in the big toe joint. There may also be crowding and rubbing of the toes. Corns can develop between the toes from the pressure of the big toe as it drifts to the side.

Bunion pain occurs for one of two reasons: *bump pain* and pain within the joint itself. Bump pain is the result of shoe pressure against the protruding, enlarged bone. With extra bone formation, the body may develop a fluid-filled sac, called a *bursa*, to protect and cushion the bone from pressure. With continued pressure on the bunion, the bursa becomes acutely inflamed and swollen, creating a painful condition called *bursitis*. Significant bump pain can also occur when a nerve adjacent to the enlarged bone becomes trapped between the bone and the shoe. Less frequently, numbness can develop over the inner top part of the big toe. Pain within the joint itself is due to altered stress inside the joint because of the abnormal position of the big toe. The cartilage on the outer side of the joint is under too much stress, leading to joint inflammation and cartilage wear, which initiate the process of arthritic change within the joint. The symptoms of bump pain versus joint pain are often hard to distinguish, although people tend to locate joint pain either around the edges of the bump or more deeply within the foot. Joint pain is often described as throbbing and aching, and patients commonly say that the pain occurs whenever they bend the toe, even when sitting. They often describe feeling like the joint needs to be cracked.

If a bunion is not painful and doesn't limit activity, you may decide not to have it treated. However, bunions usually get progressively worse over time with an increased risk of pain and joint arthritis, so some people decide to pursue treatment even if they don't have symptoms. Having the big toe in an abnormal position for a prolonged time alters the distribution of pressure within the joint. Focused pressure applied to one side of the joint can lead to thinning and deterioration of the cartilage in the joint, and worn or defective cartilage causes pain (see chapter 11). If you experience progressive and continuous pain and deformity from a bunion, we recommend that you consult a podiatrist who has had surgical training.

The only way to treat the structural problem of a bunion is with surgery. However, several nonsurgical options treat the symptoms and sometimes provide sufficient relief so that surgery isn't necessary. These options include changing to different shoes, such as shoes with a wider toe box or with soft uppers like mesh; wearing stiff-soled shoes to limit motion at the painful

joint; stretching shoes to make the toe box roomier; padding the foot to
relieve direct pressure; using toe spacers to limit rubbing between the toes; or
wearing custom-made insoles to control faulty foot mechanics. Nonsteroidal
anti-inflammatory drugs (NSAIDs) and cortisone injections directly into the
joint can be used to reduce inflammation and thereby relieve pain. If nonsurgical treatments fail to provide adequate relief from symptoms, then you
should consider surgical correction.

The goal of surgery is to eliminate pain, remove any bony prominences,
and realign the foot and joint. Surgery can also ease the symptoms of arthritis within the joint by stimulating tissue to grow and replace the normal
cartilage on the surfaces of the joint. There is no "cookbook" way to treat a
bunion surgically. The podiatrist will assess many factors, including the severity of the bunion, the condition of the big toe joint, your age, your ability
to tolerate recuperation after surgery (for example, some bunion procedures
require using crutches to keep weight off the foot for six to eight weeks),
and your expectations. There are, however, two general categories of bunion
surgery. Joint-sparing procedures involve cutting and realigning the bones
that contribute to the bunion while preserving the joint. Joint-destructive
procedures are reserved for bunions where the joint has undergone severe
degenerative changes. In these cases, preserving the joint would not provide
adequate pain relief nor address the significant damage to the joint. Therefore,
the surgery removes the arthritic joint altogether. This can be achieved by
placing soft tissue between the bones that make up the joint, by inserting
a metallic or silicone implant into the joint, or by fusing the two bones to
stiffen the joint permanently.

Bunion surgery is usually very successful, as shown in figure 8.2. How
quickly you can expect to return to walking in a normal shoe depends on
the severity of the bunion and the complexity of the surgery. In mild to
moderate cases, a patient can walk in a surgical shoe immediately, with a
return to normal shoes within six weeks. A more severe case might mean
that the patient will have to ambulate without bearing any weight for six to
eight weeks, with a return to shoes no sooner than ten to twelve weeks. As
with any surgical procedure, you should carefully consider and discuss with
your podiatrist the inherent risks and potential complications before electing

to undergo surgery. Bunions can recur after surgery; to minimize this chance, wear appropriate shoes. Custom-made orthotics can also help by addressing faulty foot mechanics.

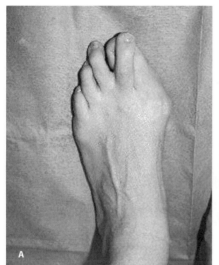 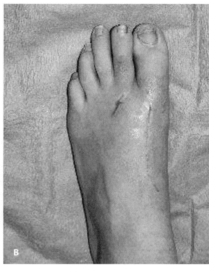

Figure 8.2. Before and after surgery to correct a classic bunion. In this case, the hammertoe (second toe) was also realigned.

Tailor's Bunion

In contrast to the classic bunion, the tailor's bunion is a painful bone enlargement on the outer edge of the foot at the base of the little toe. It is more commonly seen in women, because women generally wear tighter shoes than men. The tailor's bunion develops progressively over time, mainly due to an inherited abnormal foot structure. The mechanics of the foot are altered because the faulty structure creates bowing or splaying of the long bone, the fifth metatarsal, behind the little toe. The long bone becomes prominent on the outer edge of the front of the foot. Excess abnormal bone formation may occur at this site from external pressure, such as by tight-fitting shoes, as well as by the altered foot mechanics. Sometimes, the body responds to repetitive pressure by thickening the soft tissue and skin over the bunion, an unfortunate response that actually increases the pressure and therefore the pain.

Other causes of a tailor's bunion include trauma to the foot, inflammatory arthritis, and flexible ligaments leading to splaying of the foot bones.

Over time, a tailor's bunion may become red, swollen, and painful, although some are symptom-free. People often complain of worsening symptoms when they wear certain shoes. As with the classic bunion, non-surgical treatment of a tailor's bunion aims at reducing the symptoms rather than correcting the deformity.

Conservative options include wearing a shoe with a wider toe box or softer upper, or vamp (see chapter 3), padding the bunion or the shoe to ease the pressure, and using a custom-made orthotic to rebalance and control the faulty foot mechanics. Inflammation and pain can be treated with ice, NSAIDs, and cortisone injections.

If these nonsurgical options fail, surgical correction is a reasonable option. The goal of surgery for a tailor's bunion is to remove any bony prominences and to realign the bone structure. If you have this surgery, you can expect to return to wearing normal shoes within four to six weeks. A tailor's bunion can recur after surgery, and as with a classic bunion, the chances of recurrence are minimized by wearing appropriate shoes and possibly using an orthotic.

Bent Toes: Hammertoes, Claw Toes, and Mallet Toes

A hammertoe is any toe, other than the big toe, that bends abnormally. Hammertoes are usually flexible at first, but if they are not treated, they may become a rigid deformity. A flexible hammertoe can be fully straightened manually. A semi-rigid hammertoe can be only partially straightened, while a rigid hammertoe cannot be straightened at all. The foot has extensor tendons on the top of the toes to pull the toes up and flexor tendons on the bottom to pull the toes down. If the normal balance between the extensors and flexors is altered, the affected toes will no longer be straight. They will deform up or down or from side to side. The hammertoe condition can happen to a single toe on the foot or to several toes.

The hammertoe is the most common of three types of toe contraction that can occur. The other two are claw toes and mallet toes. All three types are shown in figure 8.3. Specifically, a hammertoe involves upward bending (extension) at both the joint at the ball of the foot (metatarsophalangeal joint) and the joint at the end of the toe (distal interphalangeal joint). The middle joint (proximal interphalangeal joint) bends down (flexion). The result is a toe that bends up in the middle. A claw toe also involves upward bending of the joint at the ball of the foot, with downward bending at both of the toe joints. Therefore, a claw toe looks like an upside down U or J. Mallet toes have downward bending at the end toe joint, and the other two joints are normal. Hammertoes, claw toes, and mallet toes all have the same causes and treatments, so for the remainder of this discussion, we refer only to hammertoes.

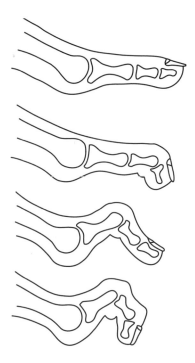

Figure 8.3. From top to bottom: normal toe, mallet toe, hammertoe, and claw toe.

   The most common factor leading to hammertoes is inheriting a foot with faulty mechanics, such as a flat foot or a high-arched foot. Over time, walking on a foot with one of these conditions causes various tendons to fire early or to work longer or harder than normal as they attempt to get the foot into a neutral position. Some of these tendons are the extensor and flexor tendons that lift and pull down the toes, and if either of these gains an advantage over other muscles in the foot, they can deform the toes. Another significant factor in developing hammertoes is wearing improper shoes. Shoes that are too shallow from top to bottom or too narrow from side to side compress the toes. Also, high-heeled shoes and shoes that are too short cramp the toes against the front of the shoe, forcing the toes into a bent position. Bunions can also force the adjacent toes into an abnormal position. Other factors that can cause hammertoes to form include neuromuscular disease, traumatic injury, inflammatory arthritis, diabetes mellitus, and stroke. The incidence of developing a hammertoe increases with age, which is consistent with the progressive nature of the problem.

Some people with hammertoes have no symptoms and are most concerned with the abnormal appearance of their affected toes. Some experience cramping of the toes or difficulty moving a hammertoe. Most people experience symptoms of pain, swelling, redness, and difficulty wearing certain shoes. The symptoms develop for various reasons. The abnormal joint in a hammertoe is more prominent than in a normal toe, resulting in pressure and irritation from shoes. A callus or corn may develop over the protruding joint and create a burning pain. (See chapter 6 for a detailed discussion of calluses and corns.) With continued pressure on a hammertoe, the soft tissue between the skin and bone may become inflamed, leading to more acute symptoms such as sharp, shooting, burning, or throbbing pain. A bursa may form underneath the callus as the body attempts to protect and cushion the affected toe, and pressure on the bursa can lead to bursitis. In addition, it is possible to develop an open wound, or ulcer, under a callus. Ulcers can cause localized redness and swelling. If you have a hammertoe, you may also experience secondary pain in the ball of the foot (see metatarsalgia, below).

Treatment of hammertoes focuses on accommodating the abnormal toe, providing relief from the symptoms, and sometimes realigning the toe surgically. Straps and splints can be used to hold a flexible hammertoe in a corrected position, thus reducing pressure from shoes. Rigid hammertoes often respond better to the use of pads, moleskin, or protective silicone or foam sleeves. These options won't fix the contracted toe; rather, they attempt to cushion the toe or maintain it in a better position. Corns and calluses should be trimmed to reduce skin thickening and to help alleviate pain. However, if you decide to trim a corn or callus at home, use extreme caution, because it is very easy to cut into the deeper skin, making the toe susceptible to bacterial infection. We recommend that anyone with a callus or corn over a hammertoe consult a podiatrist for proper paring of the thickened skin. Medicated pads or patches can be used on corns and calluses, but they also should be used cautiously (and not at all if you have diabetes or poor circulation), because they may create blisters or cause an open wound.

An orthotic may be helpful in slowing the progression of a hammertoe if you use it early in the onset of the contracted toe. Custom-made orthotics assist in controlling the faulty position and mechanics of the foot that lead to muscular imbalance within the toe. Cortisone injections can also be useful in easing symptoms of inflammation within the joints of the toe or in the soft tissues. In the past, stretching and strengthening exercises have been advocated as a hammertoe treatment, but they have not been proven effective in adults. The exercises may have some use in infants and toddlers. If you have one or several hammertoes, you should choose shoes with a low heel, a wide and deep toe box, and a soft upper material.

Surgical correction of a hammertoe is warranted if conservative treatment fails. The purpose of surgery is to realign the toe by rebalancing it with various bone and soft tissue procedures. The choice of procedure depends on the flexibility of the toe, other coexisting deformities in the foot, and the location of the imbalance. Flexible hammertoes may be best corrected with a soft tissue procedure, such as releasing tight joint ligaments and contracted tendons. If this type of procedure fails to realign the toe, the podiatrist may recommend surgically cutting and removing a small piece of bone in the contracted joint to relieve tension at the apex of the hammertoe. For more severe and rigid hammertoes, a podiatrist often recommends fusing two bones in the toe to permanently stiffen it. This bone fusion is called an *arthrodesis*. A pin is typically used to hold the fused bones together while they heal in a corrected position and is removed after four to six weeks.

If a hammertoe is contracted from side to side, as well as either up or down, additional soft tissue and bone procedures may be needed. One such bone procedure involves cutting the metatarsal bone behind the toe to relieve tension and to allow the joint at the ball of the foot to be moved into a corrected position. The toes and joint are then held in a corrected position for four to six weeks, sometimes longer, using either surgical pins or tape. You would wear a stiff-soled shoe for this period. The toe may return to its hammertoe position, so a podiatrist will often place the toe in an overcorrected position to account for some recurrence.

Pain at the Ball of the Foot: Metatarsalgia

Some people with hammertoes experience a secondary pain in the ball of the foot behind the toes, a condition known as metatarsalgia. Typically, this condition is created by excess pressure and stress to the metatarsal head behind the toes. Ideally, each of the five metatarsal heads bears weight evenly, but problems develop when one or more bear excessive weight. Depending on the pattern of weight distribution, a broad, diffuse callus may form below one or several metatarsal heads (see chapter 6 for more detail about calluses). Strictly speaking, metatarsalgia is not a toe disorder, but we include it here because of its relationship with hammertoes and bunions, both of which can contribute to an excess load on the metatarsal heads. However, it is possible to experience metatarsalgia without having hammertoes or a bunion. In fact, the condition has many other causes.

Metatarsalgia is often seen in people who participate in high-impact sports or intense training. Running, for example, creates repetitive high-pressure loading to the forefoot. Another cause is having a foot shape, such as a high arch, that overloads the front of the foot and increases stress on the metatarsal bones. As we age, the pad of fat under the metatarsals atrophies, diminishing the body's natural cushion under these bones, which may cause pain. Tight-fitting shoes and high-heeled shoes also force excessive weight onto the ball of the foot and can displace the fat pad forward so that it is no longer beneath the weight-bearing surface of the metatarsal heads. Last, a fracture or previous foot surgery that has altered the shape of the foot can contribute to increased loading on the ball of the foot.

Symptoms of metatarsalgia include aching, sharp, or burning pain in the ball of the foot. The pain is worse when standing, walking, or engaging in other weight-bearing activities, and rest relieves the discomfort. Symptoms usually develop gradually over time and become progressively worse. The skin and soft tissue in the ball of the foot underneath the metatarsals can become thickened and inflamed. Additionally, a bursa can develop as the body attempts to cushion areas receiving repetitive pressure. The bursa can give the sensation of having a rubber ball beneath the forefoot and may become inflamed and painful (bursitis).

Nonsurgical treatment of metatarsalgia addresses the symptoms. A podiatrist may recommend that you decrease your activity level to rest and relieve the pressure on your forefoot. You can get additional relief of pressure with padding to cushion the forefoot or to direct pressure off the painful site, changing shoes, or using custom-made orthotic devices to address abnormal foot mechanics and redistribute the excess weight-bearing forces on the forefoot. NSAIDs can help to reduce pain and inflammation, and in severe cases, cortisone injections may be helpful. When conservative treatments fail to alleviate symptoms, then surgery may be an option for you. Surgery must address all contributing structural deformities, with the goal of creating even pressure distribution across the front part of the foot. If a bunion or hammertoe is contributing to the problem, then it would be realigned, and the involved metatarsals would be surgically cut to elevate, shorten, or lengthen them depending on the problem. These procedures would create an even platform for the person to walk on. After surgical correction of metatarsalgia, you can typically expect four to six weeks of protected weight bearing, which means walking in a surgical shoe.

An Unstable Joint: Predislocation Syndrome

Instability of the joint at the ball of the foot, the metatarsophalangeal joint, is referred to as *predislocation syndrome*. You may also hear it referred to as *metatarsophalangeal joint capsulitis*. If left untreated, the condition can progress to total joint dislocation. Predislocation syndrome occurs most commonly in the joints behind the second, third, and fourth toes, as shown in figure 8.4A. The early signs of the condition include pain and swelling at the base of the toe, where it meets the foot, and in the toe itself. There may also be a sensation of fullness at the front of the foot. After the syndrome has progressed, the affected toe lifts up so that it might not touch the ground when the person stands, and sometimes the toe bends sideways. Hammertoes may form, and because of the sideways drift, they often overlap an adjacent toe, which is referred to as *flexor plate displacement*. Pain can occur on the top of the toe from rubbing shoes and on the adjacent toe and below the metatarsal head of the affected toe from the abnormal forces on the toe. The toe becomes irritated from rubbing against the top of the shoe. These symptoms are the result of gradual thinning, stretching, or tearing of the plantar plate ligament,

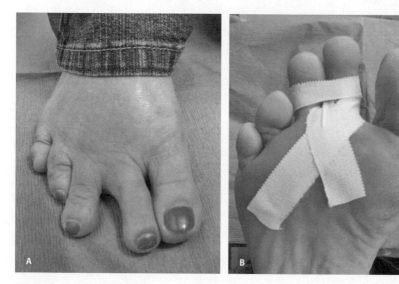

Figure 8.4. (A) Predislocation syndrome in the second toe that has progressed to flexor plate displacement. (B) Criss-cross toe taping for predislocation syndrome.

which is on the bottom of the joint. When functioning correctly, this ligament prevents the toe from lifting out of the joint.

Predislocation syndrome / flexor plate displacement is usually caused by mechanical overload or repetitive stress to the joint from activities such as repetitive stooping, squatting, and running. Heredity also makes some people more prone to this syndrome; for example, people with an exceptionally long second metatarsal bone often develop predislocation syndrome. Additional contributing factors include tight or high-heeled shoes, trauma to the forefoot, and inflammatory arthritis.

Early treatment involves taping or splinting the affected toe, as shown in figure 8.4B, to immobilize the joint. The immobilization prevents continued stretching of the plantar plate ligament, allowing the ligament to repair itself. The toe remains immobilized like this for at least four to six weeks, and sometimes longer if you can tolerate it. The taping and splinting methods also help keep the toe from rubbing on the top of your shoes. NSAIDs can be used to help reduce pain and inflammation. For more painful joints, cortisone injections can be administered. If you experience severe pain, you may find that complete immobilization of the foot is helpful. Your foot can be immobilized with a stiff-soled shoe, walking cast, or walking boot. Custom-made orthotics can also be useful to address any abnormal foot mechanics that may be contributing to the syndrome. We recommend that you get a referral to a rheumatologist to assess and treat any associated inflammatory arthritis.

You may decide to pursue surgical treatment of predislocation syndrome if nonsurgical treatments are not successful. The goal of surgery is to stabilize and realign the affected toe and joint. Surgery may consist of repairing or tightening the ligament, transferring tendons, correcting a hammertoe, or cutting the metatarsal bone behind the toe. If you have other foot conditions, such as a bunion, they may be addressed at the same time. Recuperation usually requires protected weight bearing in a stiff-soled surgical shoe for four to six weeks.

Chapter 9

Heel Pain

AT ONE TIME OR another, most adults have experienced heel pain, usually as a result of overuse. The heel takes a lot of pounding because it is the first part of the foot to contact the ground when we walk. It's also involved in transferring weight from the back to the front of the foot with each step. Heel pain occurs either on the sole (plantar) or in the back (posterior) of the heel. Pain on the sole of the heel is usually caused by structural and functional imbalances in the foot, such as a thinning fat pad under the heel bone or tension in the plantar fascia, the ligament that forms the arch. Pain in the back of the heel tends to result from a bony enlargement called Haglund's deformity or from Achilles tendonitis.

Plantar fasciitis, Haglund's deformity, and Achilles tendonitis are the three most common causes of heel pain. In this chapter, we describe the causes, symptoms, and treatment options for each one. Another heel condition, Sever disease, occurs only in children and is discussed in chapter 13.

A Strained Arch Ligament: Plantar Fasciitis

The plantar fascia is the ligament that runs from the heel bone, or calcaneus, to the base of the toes. It helps to form and stabilize the foot's arch and functions as a stress absorber. When the plantar fascia ligament is strained, it becomes inflamed and painful, a condition called *plantar fasciitis*. Just as a taut bowstring arches a bow, the plantar fascia "bows up" the arch of the foot; the ligament provides the arch with about 25 percent of its support and strength (bones, muscles, tendons, and joint ligaments provide the other 75 percent). When activities place excessive weight or force on the foot, the foot elongates and the plantar fascia flattens. This flattening increases the tension in the ligament, and it pulls on its attachment point in the heel, initiating the inflammation and pain. Plantar fasciitis occurs most commonly where the ligament attaches to the bottom of the heel bone. Less frequently, it occurs in the middle of the ligament, at the arch of the foot.

Plantar fasciitis affects people of all ages and fitness levels. It is commonly caused by prolonged walking or standing, often on hard surfaces; being overweight or rapidly gaining weight; starting a new exercise program; using improper training techniques; or wearing inappropriate or worn-down shoes. In addition, with age, the fat pad under the heel becomes thinner, decreasing the cushioning for the bottom of the heel bone. In this case, the body may form a fluid-filled sac, or bursa, to provide extra cushioning, and if it becomes inflamed, it causes bursitis. Although bursitis under the heel isn't a true fasciitis, the symptoms and treatment are similar.

Symptoms of plantar fasciitis include burning, throbbing, and aching on the inside edge or center of the heel's sole. You may experience pain on the outer edge of the heel's sole, but this pain usually develops later as a result

---

Baxter's Nerve Entrapment

Baxter's nerve is the first branch that extends off the lateral plantar nerve. This nerve syndrome's signs and symptoms directly mimic those of plantar fasciitis, so we describe this syndrome only briefly. Often, a patient whose plantar fasciitis is not responding to conservative treatment may in fact have Baxter's nerve entrapment. The diagnosis is made with nerve conduction studies, which are described in detail in chapter 10. Treatment can include nonsteroidal anti-inflammatory medication, cortisone injections, supportive taping of the arch, custom-made orthotics, and for difficult cases, immobilization in a walking cast for four to six weeks. Particularly stubborn cases require surgery to release the ligaments that are impinging on the nerve.

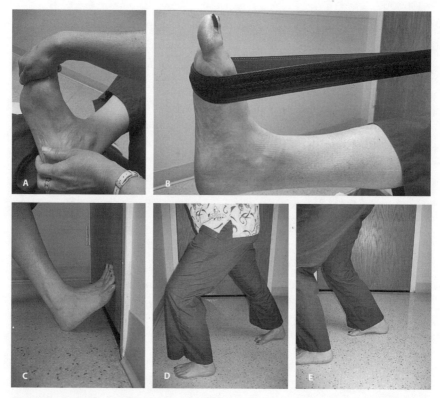

Figure 9.1. (A) Foot stretch. (B) Towel or belt stretch. (C) Wall stretch. (D) Standing calf stretch of the gastrocnemius muscle. (E) Standing calf stretch of the soleus muscle. (See the box opposite for stretching instructions.)

of walking on the outside of the heel in an effort not to place pressure on the initial site of discomfort. The pain of plantar fasciitis is often most severe immediately after resting, such as first thing in the morning. This pain results from the tearing of microscopic fibers of scar tissue that had begun to form while the foot was resting. After taking a few steps, this micro-tearing stops and the pain subsides. Prolonged activity, however, tends to increase the pain.

Treatment of plantar fasciitis aims to reduce inflammation, support the arch, and eliminate pain. The first stage in treatment generally involves taking nonsteroidal anti-inflammatory medication, wearing supportive and cushioned shoes, using over-the-counter insoles or arch supports, and modifying activity to rest the foot as much as possible. You may also find it helpful to stretch a tight calf muscle and Achilles tendon with the exercises shown in

Achilles Tendon and Plantar Fascia Stretches

Do the following stretches with both legs two or three times a day to improve the flexibility of your Achilles tendon and plantar fascia ligament.

Gastrocnemius muscle stretch: Stand about three feet away from the wall. Take a step back with the leg to be stretched and a step closer to the wall with the opposite leg. In the leg you are stretching, keep the back of the heel flat on the floor and the foot slightly turned in (adducted). Now lean your hips in toward the wall and hold the position for 30 seconds without bouncing. You should feel a pulling or tightness in the calf muscle close to the knee. Alternate legs so that the leg that was in front now goes to the back. Repeat the exercise three times for each leg.

Soleus muscle stretch: Stand as above, but bend the back knee as if to sit down on the back leg. Hold this position for 30 seconds without bouncing. You should feel a pulling or tightness in the back of the leg close to the ankle. Alternate legs and repeat three times for each leg.

Plantar fascia ligament stretch: Sit on a chair and bring one leg up and over to rest the outer ankle on the knee of the other leg. With one hand, gently pull the toes as far as they can go toward the shin. You should feel the stretch on the bottom of the foot. You can also do this stretch using a belt or standing against a wall.

figure 9.1. If these treatments prove ineffective, then the next stage is to try cortisone injections to relieve pain and inflammation, custom-made orthotics, physical therapy, and night splints that are designed to help with stretching the plantar fascia. When the plantar fasciitis is not responding well to this line of treatment, it may be necessary to immobilize the foot for four to six weeks in a CAM walking cast (usually referred to as a CAM walker). Full recovery from plantar fasciitis can take six to twelve months with these conservative treatments. If they fail to work, then other options can be considered, but we

strongly recommend trying to resolve the condition with conservative treatments for at least a six-month period.

More invasive treatment options include shock wave therapy (high-energy
shock waves guided by ultrasound to stimulate repair of the plantar fascia
where it attaches to the heel), endoscopic plantar fasciotomy (making a small
incision to release tension in part of the plantar fascia), and open surgery
(cutting the ligament, as above, and removing a heel spur, if present).

We recommend that you wear an orthotic after treatment until the heel is
completely pain-free, and if you spend a lot of time on your feet every day,
it would be wise to wear an orthotic indefinitely to minimize the chance
of recurrence. Once the pain is gone or only mild symptoms remain, you
can gradually increase your level of activity. Plantar fasciitis may recur once
treated, and sometimes it will occur in the other heel while the treated heel
remains free of pain.

A Bump on the Heel: Haglund's Deformity

A harmless but painful bony enlargement on the outer posterior heel is
called a Haglund's deformity, seen in figure 9.2, named for the doctor who
first described it. This condition is commonly referred to as a "pump bump,"
because women's pump-style shoes, with rigid heel counters, contribute to
its symptoms. Given this common name, it isn't surprising that Haglund's
deformity occurs most frequently in women who spend a lot of time wearing dress shoes.

Most people with Haglund's deformity have inherited a foot structure
with this bony enlargement present at birth. With pressure and rubbing on
the heel over time, a bursa forms and becomes inflamed and painful (bursitis). High-arched feet, in particular, tend to supinate when walking (inward
movement of the heel causing a person to walk on the outside of the heel),
causing the back of the heel to rub repetitively against the shoe's heel counter. A tight or shortened Achilles tendon also contributes to the condition by
compressing another bursa (the retrocalcaneal bursa, which everybody has)
against the heel bone. Symptoms of Haglund's deformity include pain, redness, and swelling at the back of the heel. Often, a callus also develops over
the affected area.

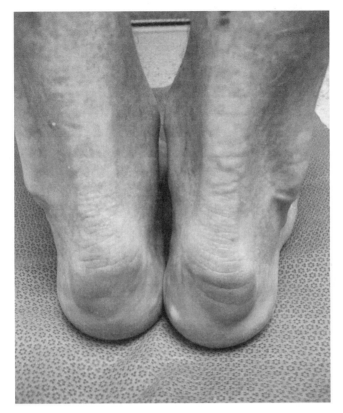

Figure 9.2. Haglund's deformity is a bony enlargement on the back of the heel.

Treatment of a Haglund's deformity begins with taking nonsteroidal anti-inflammatory medications, switching to open-back shoes, inserting heel lifts into shoes to elevate the painful area away from the heel counter, and using heel pads or sleeves to protect the area. Regularly doing exercises to stretch the Achilles tendon, as shown in figure 9.1, can also be beneficial, but the exercises take time to produce results. If your symptoms don't respond to these treatments, you can try a custom-made orthotic to control supination of the foot. Physical therapy may also be helpful. If you have significant discomfort, you may need to immobilize the foot for four to six weeks. Surgery should only be considered when the symptoms don't respond to conservative treatment. The procedure usually involves removing both the prominent bony enlargement on the back of the heel bone and the inflamed bursa.

Strong, Yet Weak: Achilles Tendonitis

The Achilles tendon at the back of the lower leg and heel provides the necessary power to push the heel off the ground and transfer weight forward when we walk. The tendon is remarkably strong; it can withstand forces up to twenty thousand pounds! When the tendon is damaged, though, the result is a painful condition called *Achilles tendonitis*. Though some may blame Achilles's mother, Thetis, for poor technique at the River Styx, the Achilles tendon's susceptibility to injury stems from the relatively small blood supply that it receives at the point where it inserts into the back of the heel.

People at greatest risk of developing Achilles tendonitis are poorly conditioned "weekend warriors," although it can occur in high-level athletes, too. Improper conditioning or training and trying to do too much too soon put people at risk of damaging tendons in general. Factors that increase the risk of developing Achilles tendonitis include loss of flexibility and lack of strength in either the lower or upper leg, hill training, long-term overpronation of the foot, and wearing high-heeled shoes frequently. Sudden stress from falling down, stepping in a hole, or stepping off a curb can also damage the Achilles tendon. In addition, Achilles tendonitis can develop with repetitive stress exerted on the tendon from sports, exercise, and being on your feet all day.

Achilles tendonitis can be either acute, where the tendon becomes inflamed, or chronic, where the tendon degenerates. The acute form causes swelling and redness on the back of the heel, and pain occurs during or following activity. You may also have a sensation of creaking along the tendon, which is called *crepitus* and feels like a slight popping, clicking, or grating. The chronic form, more correctly called *tendinosis*, causes a dull ache in the back of the heel or ankle. With tendinosis, you may experience morning stiffness and pain after resting. Tendinosis involves loss of structure within the tendon, and small tears and scarring sometimes occur. This chronic degeneration causes decreased blood flow to the tendon, diminishing its ability to heal. At the point where the Achilles tendon inserts into the back of the heel, abnormal calcium deposits can form a bony outgrowth, or spur, referred to as a *retrocalcaneal exostosis* (literally, back heel spur).

Initial treatment of Achilles tendonitis is similar to the treatments previously described for plantar fasciitis and Haglund's deformity. It's often necessary to discontinue physical activity and rest the foot. Additional treatments include the use of heel lifts, heel cups, and heel sleeves for protection, as well as stretching exercises, shown in figure 9.1. If you have severe pain or the tendonitis is unresponsive to treatment, your foot may need to be immobilized in a CAM walker or non-weight-bearing hard cast for four to six weeks. Physical therapy may also be necessary for particularly stubborn cases. Surgery is reserved for tendonitis that doesn't improve with at least six months of conservative care. The surgical procedure depends on the specific location of the tendonitis, as well as the extent of degeneration, which is often determined first by magnetic resonance imaging (MRI). X-rays are also taken to evaluate for bone spurs. Typically, surgery involves removing damaged areas and repairing the tendon, as well as removing bone spurs if they are present. Recovery requires staying off the foot for four to six weeks, followed by wearing a walking boot or cast for an additional two to four weeks. You can then return to wearing a supportive shoe.

You will need physical therapy to build up strength in both the repaired tendon and the muscles that have weakened with lack of use. Physical therapy also increases the range of motion in the ankle and foot and helps to improve balance. Improving balance, or balance re-education, is necessary because both the initial tendon injury and the subsequent surgery can interrupt the body's position and balance mechanism, called *proprioception*. Tiny nerve receptors surround the joints and automatically provide the brain with information about the position of the foot and ankle. Following trauma, this position feedback mechanism is often diminished or lost, so patients are at increased risk for re-injury.

Preventing Achilles tendonitis from recurring—or from occurring in the first place—requires proper conditioning for activities. It is wise to gradually increase training intensity, stretch and strengthen the calf muscles, wear cushioned and supportive shoes, and cross-train with low-impact activities such as cycling or swimming.

Other Sources of Heel Pain

Although the three conditions described above are the most common sources of heel pain, there are a few other causes. Severe pain with every step may be the result of a stress fracture in the heel bone, discussed in more detail in chapter 14. The sensation of pins and needles or tingling may be due to tarsal tunnel syndrome, which is discussed in chapter 10, or to Baxter's nerve entrapment (see the first box in this chapter).

If you have heel pain that is not responding to the types of treatment described in this chapter, you may have a systemic (affecting the whole body) condition, such as rheumatoid arthritis, Reiter syndrome, ankylosing spondylitis, psoriatic arthritis, or gout. All of these conditions have been reported as a source of heel pain. If you have a known history for systemic arthritis, your heel pain needs to be addressed with that systemic condition in mind. In this case, the symptoms are usually not isolated to the heel. Treatments are often similar to those already described for heel pain, but you would also be referred to a rheumatologist. See chapter 11 for more details.

Chapter 10

Nerve Syndromes Affecting the Foot and Ankle

NERVES ARE THE ELECTRICAL wires of the body's peripheral nervous system. The peripheral nervous system connects the brain and spinal cord to the organs and limbs, including, of course, the feet. Just like electrical wires, nerves have an inner portion that conducts the nerve signal and an outer insulating layer. The inner portion consists of either *sensory fibers*, which allow us to feel sensations like pressure, pain, temperature, and texture, or *motor fibers*, which control the movement of muscles. (A third type of fiber controls involuntary responses within the body, such as the "fight or flight" response, heart rate, blood pressure, stimulation of the digestive system, and temperature regulation.) Because the nerves of the peripheral nervous system aren't as well protected by bone or other barriers as the spine and brain are, the peripheral nerves are at risk of being entrapped or compressed. In this chapter, we discuss several of the most common nerve syndromes that affect the foot and ankle. Figure 10.1 shows the broad areas served by the nerves that go to the lower leg and foot. Symptoms are not always isolated to this part of the body, but we focus on how the conditions directly impact the foot and ankle.

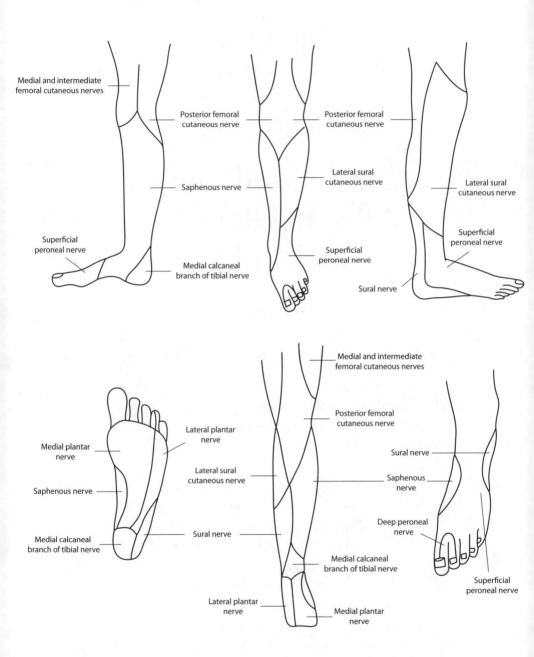

Figure 10.1. Broad areas where nerves supply the lower leg and foot.

Trapped Nerves in the Lower Back

When the roots of nerves in the lower back are compressed or subjected to excess pressure, a syndrome called *lumbosacral radiculopathy* occurs. The nerve roots emerge from between the vertebrae (bones surrounding the spinal cord). Between each vertebra lies a disc that cushions and protects the nerve roots. If one of the discs receives trauma, degenerates, or herniates (the disc extrudes through the ligaments surrounding the spine), the nerve roots can become compressed. The discs in the lower back are at particular risk of injury and herniation because of the significant amount of force they are exposed to as the human body rotates, flexes, extends, and bends from side to side. Nerves in the lower back can also be irritated by degenerative arthritis of the spine. This condition can create bone spurs and narrow the bony tunnels in which the nerves travel, causing irritation, inflammation, and swelling. If the condition affects any of the nerves in the lower back that provide sensation and muscle control to the lower leg and foot, symptoms will occur in the foot or ankle.

With a condition called *lumbosacral radiculopathy*, sensory symptoms are experienced more often than motor symptoms and generally include numbness, tingling, burning, and shooting pain; the intensity of these symptoms can vary from day to day. Pain can range from dull and difficult to pinpoint to sharp and easy to demarcate. The affected area can also be hypersensitive to the touch, a symptom known as *allodynia*. The specific part of the lower leg and foot that is affected depends on which nerve roots are compressed. For example, sciatica is a radiculopathy of one of the nerves in the lower lumbar region (medically labeled as nerve L_5), which causes pain that radiates to the buttocks and down into the leg and foot (the sciatic nerve originates from five nerve roots: L_4, L_5, S_1, S_2, and S_3).

In more advanced cases of lumbosacral radiculopathy, the muscles of the foot and ankle can become weak, and if untreated, the nerve damage and muscle weakness may be permanent. The most common foot and ankle condition associated with the muscular effects of radiculopathy is drop foot. Drop foot occurs with weakness in the muscles and tendons that lift the foot up. These muscles also decelerate the foot as it contacts the ground, converting from the swing phase to the contact phase of the gait cycle. Therefore, if you walk with a drop foot, your foot slaps down as it contacts the ground, and you may trip as you attempt to lift the foot off the ground (see chapter 4).

If you go to a physician with the type of symptoms described above, you will likely undergo several tests to determine which nerves are involved. A basic test is the straight leg raise test: you lie flat on your back and the physician elevates your leg at the hip while the knee stays straight. This position increases tension in the nerve roots and elicits pain if a root is compressed. Likewise, bending the knee during this test lessens the pain. You may go for medical imaging tests, such as x-ray and magnetic resonance imaging (MRI), to identify a herniated disc or other changes to normal anatomy. Another type of testing you may encounter is noninvasive electrodiagnostic testing, which includes nerve conduction studies and quantitative sensory testing, both of which test how well a nerve is functioning. Nerve conduction studies involve putting electrodes on the skin and stimulating a nerve with electrical impulses. Quantitative sensory testing assesses your response to light touch and to vibration. Additional testing that you may have is called electromyography, which examines the electrical activity within skeletal muscle. This test is slightly more invasive than the others because a needle electrode goes through the skin into the underlying muscle.

Treatment for lower back nerve entrapment syndromes typically starts with physical therapy, which includes lumbar strengthening, ultrasound, massage, and electrical stimulation. Rest and nonsteroidal anti-inflammatory medications are also initial treatments. (Note that *complete bed rest* is no longer considered an effective treatment for back pain. You should continue to move around unless your doctor advises you not to.) Lumbar supports or braces stabilize the spine and assist you with pain relief, while muscle relaxants can help if you experience severe spasms. Cortisone injections can be given around the affected nerve roots to provide relief of symptoms, but these injections must be done by neurosurgeons, orthopedic surgeons, or anesthesiologists who specialize in pain management. Spinal surgery is an option if you are severely limited by pain or have significant weakness in the lower limbs. This surgery targets a degenerated or herniated disc and associated arthritis.

Foot or ankle weakness that results from a lower back nerve entrapment can be treated with bracing and physical therapy. Over-the-counter and custom-made ankle braces are used to enable you to walk more easily and with a gait that is closer to normal, as well as to provide stability to the foot and ankle. If braces don't help, there are surgical options. Surgical procedures to address muscle weakness and instability include transferring unaffected tendons to other locations in the foot to assist the tendons affected by the nerve entrapment and fusing unstable joints to create a stable platform on which to walk.

Injury to the Outer Layer of a Nerve: Peripheral Neuropathy

When the outer insulating layer of a nerve becomes damaged, the condition is called a *peripheral neuropathy*. This condition can involve a single nerve or many nerves at once. Damage to a single nerve (*mononeuropathy*) can be the result of an injury or compression to the nerve, and the effects are localized to the specific part of the body where the nerve goes. Damage to more than one nerve (*polyneuropathy*) can be caused by an extremely wide range of disorders and conditions, including diabetes, anemia, inflammatory arthritis, poor circulation, kidney failure, infection (such as Lyme disease), HIV, lupus, and scleroderma. Other causes of polyneuropathy are cancer, chemotherapy, trauma to nerves, hereditary neurological conditions (for example, Friedreich ataxia, Charcot-Marie-Tooth disease), alcoholism, vitamin deficiency, and exposure to heavy metals (like lead, arsenic, mercury, gold, or silver). Last, polyneuropathy can occur when nerves are compressed by a tight cast or brace, by sitting with the legs crossed, or by lying in one position for a prolonged period, such as during a long surgical operation. The effects of a polyneuropathy tend to be more general, affecting many areas of the body.

Peripheral neuropathy can cause sensory or motor symptoms, although sensory symptoms are more common. They begin gradually with numbness, tingling, burning, and pain that can be sharp, jabbing, and electric. The pain is often worse at night, when the brain is not being simultaneously bombarded with input from the other senses—sight, sound, vision, taste, and smell. Symptoms usually begin in the toe and extend up the leg. Patients often report the sensation of wearing a sock or walking on a bunched-up sock. Other symptoms include uncoordination, loss of balance, and hypersensitivity to touch. When motor dysfunction occurs, the muscles become wasted,

or atrophied. The muscles controlled by the affected nerve become weak or
paralyzed, and they may cramp or twitch. The foot and ankle can change
structurally as the unaffected muscles overpower the weaker muscles, causing
the foot to point inward or outward, and possibly up or down.

A physician diagnoses peripheral neuropathy by taking a complete medical history and conducting a physical examination to assess sensation, reflexes,
and muscle strength in the lower leg and foot. You may also undergo noninvasive electrodiagnostic testing, as described for lower back nerve entrapment.
If you have a known condition or situation that could be contributing to
the neuropathy, the physician will determine if it's under adequate control.
For example, it is essential to control blood sugar in a person with diabetes,
provide vitamin B12 to a person with pernicious anemia, and stop alcohol
consumption by a person with alcoholism.

The damage to nerves is often progressive and permanent, so treatment
of peripheral neuropathy aims to control the symptoms, increase your ability to function independently, and prevent injury or further injury to the
lower limb. The treatment differs depending on the cause of the neuropathy.
Pharmacological treatment assists in pain relief and diminishes uncomfortable sensations such as numbness and tingling. Topical (applied to the skin)
therapies have few, if any, systemic side effects and are often very helpful. For
example, you may find relief by applying capsaicin cream three to four times
daily. One of the essential ingredients is cayenne pepper, so during about the
first two weeks of use, you will experience a burning until the skin becomes
desensitized. Topical 5 percent lidocaine patches contain a local anesthetic
(numbing agent). You can use the patches for twelve hours per day on the area
of greatest discomfort—although they must not by applied on broken skin.
Oral medication is also an option: some anticonvulsant and antidepressant
medications (for example, Neurontin, Lyrica, Cymbalta, Elavil) can effectively relieve sensory symptoms, and narcotic medication can be taken for
pain, although its use is recommended only if prescribed under the care of a
physician who specializes in pain management. Vitamin supplements, such as
vitamin B12, thiamine, and folate, may also help with symptoms, particularly
when the neuropathy is related to vitamin deficiency or alcoholism.

Physical therapy can ease the pain associated with peripheral neuropathy.
It can also assist in muscle strengthening and control. For example, electric

stimulation helps to maintain muscle tone, and ultrasound and massage aid in reducing inflammation and scarring around affected nerves. If the neuropathy includes muscle weakness in the feet, braces and custom-made orthotics can improve your ability to walk.

A final and important aspect of treatment for peripheral neuropathy is protecting the foot and lower leg to keep them safe from injury. Loss of sensation in the lower limb increases the risk of injury. Either you or someone helping you should inspect the feet and ankles daily for open wounds, redness, and swelling. Also, evaluate any surfaces that you intend to walk on or put your feet on for extremes in temperature; wear protective shoes and insoles whenever possible (see chapter 15). If you have loss of feeling in your feet and legs as well as some loss of muscle control, you may find it much easier to walk if you use a cane or walker.

It Happens in the Foot, Too: Tarsal Tunnel Syndrome

Tarsal tunnel syndrome occurs when the tibial nerve becomes trapped at the ankle, or if one of its branches into the foot becomes trapped. The tibial nerve travels down the back of the leg, behind and beneath the inside anklebone, and then into the *tarsal tunnel*. The tarsal tunnel has a floor composed of two bones, the ankle (talus) and calcaneus (heel) bones, and a ligament for its roof. From the tarsal tunnel, the tibial nerve splits into two branches that supply sensation and motor control to muscles within the foot. Because it lies within a tunnel with little room for expansion, the tibial nerve and its branches are susceptible to compression and tension.

Tarsal tunnel syndrome has multiple causes. Anything that creates swelling or takes up space within the tarsal tunnel can cause nerve entrapment. For example, a soft tissue mass, thickening or swelling around or within adjacent tendons, or varicose veins can all result in tibial nerve entrapment. Some systemic diseases, including rheumatoid arthritis and other inflammatory arthritides, diabetes, and hypothyroidism, can create swelling around or within the nerve. Trauma that creates scar tissue around the nerve and bony prominences or spurs that apply pressure to the nerve can both lead to tarsal tunnel syndrome. The flatfoot condition also increases tension on the tibial nerve. Last, there is the *double crush phenomenon*, whereby multiple nerve entrapments occur simultaneously. For example, when nerve compression or damage occurs higher in the body than the foot or ankle, such as in the lower back, nerve cells in the leg, foot, and ankle become more susceptible to compression.

The symptoms of tarsal tunnel syndrome are numbness, tingling, burning, and a feeling of getting electric shocks in the region of the tibial nerve around the inside of the ankle, heel, arch, sole of the foot, and bottom of the toes. Sometimes, a pins-and-needles sensation extends up the leg or into the foot. Discomfort is usually made worse by increased activity, such as walking or prolonged standing, and is relieved with rest, elevation, or massage.

Tarsal tunnel syndrome can be identified by a doctor who tests for a tingling sensation in the sole of the foot or toes when the tibial nerve is tapped. This sensation is referred to as a positive Tinel's sign. You may have electrodiagnostic testing, as described earlier in this chapter, to confirm the diagnosis. MRI can also be helpful to determine whether there are tumors within the tarsal tunnel, abnormalities of the adjacent tendons, or varicose veins. Your physician may also send you to have blood drawn to determine if you have any contributing systemic conditions, such as inflammatory arthritis, diabetes, thyroid disease, or vitamin insufficiency.

Treatment of tarsal tunnel syndrome depends on the cause. If a flat foot has contributed to nerve tension, then the faulty mechanics of the foot are addressed with supportive shoes, arch supports, or custom-made orthotics. Rest and immobilization can also reduce your symptoms. If varicose veins are to blame, compression stockings can alleviate vein engorgement. If tendonitis or scar tissue is the cause, physical therapy might be helpful. Cortisone injections around the nerve can assist in reducing pain.

If your symptoms don't respond to conservative approaches, and if you have an identifiable soft tissue mass or bone spur within the tarsal tunnel, we recommend surgery. The procedure releases the tight ligament that forms the roof of the tunnel and removes any soft tissues or bony lesions that are occupying space in the tarsal tunnel. Any tendon swelling or thickening is also addressed by releasing fibrous structures around the nerve or by opening the nerve and cleaning it of scar tissue. After surgery, you will not be allowed to bear weight on the foot for two to four weeks and can then gradually return to full weight bearing in a normal shoe. Faulty foot mechanics should continue to be addressed after surgery with custom-made orthotics.

Injury to Nerves that Serve the Toes: Morton's Neuroma

Morton's neuroma describes an entrapment of one of the *intermetatarsal nerves*, which supply nerve signals to the toes. Although any of the nerves supplying the toes can be affected, Morton's neuroma occurs most commonly with the nerve that supplies the outside of the third toe and inside of the fourth toe. This nerve has little freedom to move and is therefore susceptible to repetitive compression, pressure, and tension, which create scarring, thickening, and swelling around and within the nerve. The word *neuroma* means "benign tumor on a nerve," but for Morton's neuroma, the name is misleading because no tumor is involved; instead, the nerve is entrapped by the formation of fibrous tissue within and surrounding it. Morton's neuroma affects women more often than men.

Direct compression or tension on the nerve may irritate it. Flat feet (see chapter 5) are considered a cause of Morton's neuroma both by increasing tension along the digital nerves with outward movement of the foot and by creating shearing forces beneath the metatarsal heads. Also, greater mobility of the metatarsals may irritate the intermetatarsal nerves. Tight or high-heeled shoes can contribute to neuroma formation by squeezing the metatarsal heads together, which compresses the nerves, and by excessively loading the ball of the foot, which places direct pressure on the nerves between the metatarsal heads. Wearing a high-heeled shoe can also place tension on these nerves by forcing the toes to hyperextend. This hyperextension not only stretches the nerve, but pulls it taut against an overlying ligament, leading to irritation. Toe hyperextension can also be seen with hammertoes (see chapter 8). Another cause of a Morton's neuroma is direct trauma to the nerve from activities such as running and racquet sports, which transmit repetitive forces to the ball of the foot.

With a Morton's neuroma, you experience pain that can range from dull to sharp at the place where the nerve is trapped between the metatarsal heads and extending into the affected toes. The pain becomes worse when standing and when wearing shoes, particularly high heels. You may feel burning, numbness, tingling, and cramping in the toes, although it is unusual to lose all sensation. People with Morton's neuroma often report the feeling of walking on a pebble or marble, as well as having the urge to massage the ball of the foot.

A podiatrist will usually diagnose a Morton's neuroma with physical examination, including an easy test called Mulder's sign, which mimics what happens in the foot with weight bearing. The test involves using one hand to pinch the skin and soft tissues between the two affected toes and the other hand to squeeze the sides of the foot together. Doing so when Morton's neuroma is present usually produces a clicking sensation, which both you and the physician will feel. Other diagnostic tests you may encounter are x-rays, MRI, and high-resolution ultrasound.

Treatment of a Morton's neuroma begins with trying to eliminate pressure or tension on the nerve and relieving the pain and inflammation. We recommend that you rest and reduce the amount of time spent in weight-bearing activities. Taking nonsteroidal anti-inflammatory medication also helps. If a flatfoot condition is involved, you can ease tension on the nerve by wearing an over-the-counter or custom-made arch support. Pads applied to shoe insoles or arch supports just behind the ball of the foot can stabilize and separate the metatarsals, thereby dispersing pressure away from the neuroma. With Morton's neuroma, you will likely find it beneficial to wear supportive and cushioned shoes with a wide toe box and a thick rubber sole. Avoid wearing a shoe with a heel, even a low heel, because these shoes have very little cushioning and no arch support, and they push the weight forward to the area where Morton's neuroma forms. Cortisone injections given around the nerve can reduce inflammation and also assist in reducing scar tissue. Only a limited number of cortisone injections should be given, however, because too much cortisone administered between the metatarsals leads to thinning of the fat pad under the ball of the foot.

For a Morton's neuroma that does not improve with the treatments described above, more invasive options are available. One is to inject a dilute alcohol solution around the nerve, behind the area of maximum tenderness. Generally, four to seven injections are needed, with one injection every seven to ten days. The nerve absorbs the alcohol and becomes deadened, or *sclerosed*, so that it no longer functions. Another option is radiofrequency treatment: With a local anesthetic in the area around the nerve, electrodes are inserted between the metatarsals to create an electrical field next to the neuroma. The electrical field destroys nerve tissue and relieves pain. A third option is cryogenic neuroablation, also called cryoanalgesia, which delivers a small amount of gas into the tissues around the neuroma. The gas freezes and destroys nerve tissue. Any treatment that destroys nerve tissue will permanently remove all sensation in the affected toes.

There are two main surgical options for treating Morton's neuroma: neurectomy and external neurolysis. Neurectomy involves cutting out the enlarged portion of the nerve and allowing it to retract into the muscles between the metatarsals. The nerve can then regenerate in an area that is not weight bearing and where there is little chance for tension to develop within the nerve. This surgical technique minimizes the possibility of the nerve regrowing into scar tissue; if the nerve does regrow into scar tissue, it may become trapped (referred to as stump neuroma), which can be as uncomfortable as the original condition. After surgery, you will have a four-to-six-week period of protected weight bearing in a stiff-soled shoe. You may be able to switch to sneakers or runners within three to four weeks.

External neurolysis involves freeing the affected nerve, usually from the intermetatarsal ligament, without severing the nerve itself. This surgery can be performed by cutting open the foot or by using endoscopic equipment. Again, you will be allowed to walk with protected weight bearing immediately after surgery and return to normal shoes within four to six weeks.

Other Nerve Entrapment Syndromes

Several other nerves to the lower leg and foot can also become trapped. These nerves are the common *peroneal nerve* and its two branches, the superficial and deep peroneal nerves, as well as the sural nerve. The *superficial peroneal nerve* (and its subsequent branches) supplies sensation to the top of the foot, the inside of the forefoot, and the inside and outside of most of the small toes. The *deep peroneal nerve* supplies the tissues between the big toe and the second toe, as well as the extensor muscles and tendons. The *sural nerve* supplies the outer and back sides of the lower leg, ankle, and foot.

Common Peroneal Nerve

The common peroneal nerve travels around the outside of the knee joint, so it is susceptible to injury from sitting with crossed legs for long periods, improper positioning of the leg against an operating room table during long surgeries, compressing the leg of a bedridden patient against the bed or bed rail, or having a cast on the lower leg. Other causes are soft tissue tumors, bone tumors, knee deformities, and systemic diseases such as diabetes. Common peroneal nerve entrapment can also result from trauma, including dislocating the knee, spraining the ankle where the foot turns inward, or fracturing the upper portion of the outside leg bone (fibula), which results in bone fragments compressing the nerve. People with high-arched feet tend to walk with the heel in an inverted position, which can also stretch and cause tension in the nerve.

Entrapment of the common peroneal nerve creates burning, tingling, numbness, or a pins-and-needles sensation on the front and outside of the lower leg, as well as on the top and outside of the foot and ankle. The muscles that bring the foot up and out can become weak, making it difficult to lift the foot off the ground when taking a step forward. To avoid stumbling, people typically use the thigh muscles to lift the entire leg high off the ground, producing a characteristic *steppage gait*. People with this muscle weakness may also have trouble slowing or easing the foot down as it contacts the ground, a condition referred to as a *foot slap*.

A podiatrist may recommend electrodiagnostic testing as well as x-rays and MRI, to evaluate the source of nerve compression and to recommend an appropriate treatment, which depends on the severity of the condition and the underlying cause. The first step is to eliminate the source of pressure or tension on the nerve. In the case of external pressure, the nerve often recovers and the symptoms resolve by simply removing the source of pressure. The podiatrist may recommend that you support your foot and ankle with temporary bracing or immobilization when walking to help the nerve to recover. If you have a high-arched foot that contributes to the problem, you can wear a custom-made orthotic to reposition the foot and release tension on the nerve. Nonsteroidal anti-inflammatory medication, medications such as Neurontin or Elavil, or a cortisone injection relieves inflammation and pain.

You may also undergo physical therapy to help reduce swelling or scar tissue surrounding the nerve as well as to recondition and strengthen the muscles.

Common peroneal entrapment syndromes that do not respond to conservative treatment as well as entrapments caused by soft tissue or bone lesions compressing the nerve require surgical attention. Surgery involves removing any contributing soft tissue or abnormal bone and releasing any constricting fibrous bands that overlie the nerve. Only very rarely does the nerve have to be completely removed, or excised. We recommend that you stay off the leg until the surgical stitches heal. The nerve itself takes several months to heal, provided there was no permanent damage.

Peroneal Nerves and Sural Nerve

The superficial and deep peroneal nerves and the sural nerve can all be treated in the same way to relieve the compression and symptoms from nerve entrapment. However, the causes and symptoms differ for each nerve. Here, we first describe the causes and symptoms of nerve entrapment for each of these nerves, followed by a combined discussion of treatment for these entrapment syndromes.

The superficial peroneal nerve branches from the common peroneal nerve, travels down the outside of the lower leg, and comes close to the surface under the skin above the ankle. It then splits into two branches, one that supplies nerve signals to the top and inside one-third of the foot and the big toe and one that supplies the central one-third of the top of the foot and the tops and sides of the four small toes. Where the superficial peroneal nerve comes close to the skin surface, it becomes susceptible to injury and entrapment, as do its two branches. Causes of entrapment include tight shoes or boots, bone spurs or soft tissue masses that press on the nerve at the front of the ankle and top of the foot, trauma or bruising to the front of the leg or top of the foot, and ankle sprains that stretch the nerve. A high-arched foot with an inverted heel can also place tension on the nerve. The two branches of the superficial peroneal nerve are also vulnerable to injury or entrapment during ankle surgery. Symptoms include a sharp or burning pain at the point where the nerve is trapped, loss of sensation to light touch at the front of the ankle and on top of the foot and toes (although you may still have pain, even with this loss of sensation), and tingling when the nerve is tapped (Tinel's sign).

The deep peroneal nerve also branches from the common peroneal nerve, travels along the front of the lower leg to the top of the middle of the foot, and then supplies sensation between the big toe and the second toe. Deep peroneal nerve entrapment (also called anterior tarsal tunnel syndrome) most commonly occurs in the front of the ankle and in the two locations where the nerve is near the skin surface, which are on the outside of the leg just below the knee and on the top of the foot. The nerve can be entrapped by direct trauma to the upper leg or middle of the foot, soft tissue or bone tumors, bone spurs, tight or high-heeled shoes, and a foot position with the heel turned inward. Kneeling with the top of the foot flat on the floor and the legs underneath the weight of the body stretches the nerve. Inflammation or thickening of the tendons adjacent to the nerve can also compress it. Your symptoms may include pain, tingling, burning, and loss of sensation between the first and second toe. Often, tingling is worse with tight shoes or boots, and moving the ankle can exacerbate the symptoms. Weakness in the muscles that lift the foot, and the resultant "foot drop," occur with longstanding compression of the nerve at the top of the lower leg.

The sural nerve begins in the back of the calf, travels along the outside of the Achilles tendon, and then runs along the outside of the foot and ankle. It supplies feeling to the back and outside of the lower leg and the outside of the heel and foot. Causes of sural nerve entrapment include direct trauma to the nerve, ankle sprains that stretch the nerve, soft tissue masses and bone spurs along its course, and thickening of tendons, including the Achilles tendon, alongside the nerve. Scarring from prior surgery and broken bones can also impinge on or damage the sural nerve. You may experience symptoms of pain, tingling, and numbness in the outer foot and ankle, calf pain, and possible sensory loss along the length of the nerve. Symptoms usually are made worse as you increase your level of activity and when you try to turn your foot inward.

For all of these nerve entrapment syndromes, treatment should begin by wearing different shoes or using custom-made orthotics to try to eliminate or minimize tension on and compression of the nerve. You can take nonsteroidal anti-inflammatory medication and have cortisone injections to alleviate the pain and swelling. Cortisone injections can also help to diminish scar tissue surrounding the nerve. If your nerve syndrome doesn't respond to these conservative measures, surgery is an option. A podiatrist may begin with some of the minimally invasive surgical options discussed under Morton's neuroma, including dilute alcohol injections, radiofrequency, and cryoanalgesia. These procedures can be used provided there is no bone or soft tissue lesion compressing the nerve. Surgery releases constricting fibrous structures and removes soft tissue masses or bone spurs at the point where they impinge or compress the nerve. If it is significantly damaged, from direct trauma, for example, the podiatrist may perform a neurectomy to cut the nerve and bury it or to allow it to retract into the surrounding muscles.

Chapter 11

Arthritis Affecting Foot and Ankle Joints

THE WORD *arthritis* means inflammation (*-itis*) of a joint (*arthro*). Healthy joints move smoothly, and in feet and ankle joints, they help with shock absorption. However, when one or more of the components of a joint—cartilage, ligament, tendon, or capsule—are damaged, the joint loses stability and no longer moves smoothly. A damaged joint, no matter the exact cause of the damage, is arthritic. Arthritis can affect any joint in the body, and it can be painful, limiting, and disabling. Regardless of the location of an arthritic joint, the causes, symptoms, diagnosis, and treatment are similar. This chapter discusses the three most common forms of arthritis that affect the joints of the foot and ankle: osteoarthritis, rheumatoid arthritis, and gout.

Worn Cartilage: Osteoarthritis

Osteoarthritis describes the wearing down of cartilage within a joint. Cartilage is the tissue that protects and cushions bones while the joint moves. Cartilage can deteriorate and become thinner, either uniformly or in sections, causing the bones to lose their protective coating and smooth gliding surface. The loss of cartilage means that within the joint, there are areas where bone rubs on bone. Despite being rigid and seemingly fixed, bones are continuously going through a process called *remodeling*, in which old bone is removed (*resorption*) and new bone is formed (*ossification*). Bone remodeling is one reason that a fracture heals.

With persistent rubbing, bone formation lays down a thicker layer underneath the area of worn cartilage, called a *subchondral sclerosis*. X-rays pick up this thicker layer as a dense white area within the bone just below the cartilage, as seen in figure 11.1. Extra bone may also form in areas around the periphery of the joint as the body attempts to redistribute the weight and associated forces borne by the joint by increasing the surface area within the joint. These extra growths of bone are termed bone spurs, or *osteophytes*.

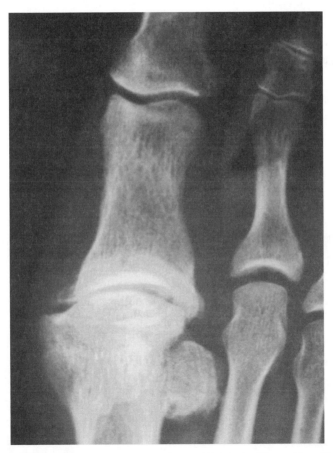

Figure 11.1. In the toe with osteoarthritis, dense white bone is visible on either side of the joint. There is uneven narrowing of the joint space in the toe on the left, compared with the normal joint space in the toe to the right.

As the osteoarthritis progresses, fluid-filled cysts may form within the bone beneath areas where the cartilage has eroded. With continued loss of joint cartilage, the joint may become narrower (the distance from bone to bone becomes shorter), as seen in figure 11.1. Loose pieces of cartilage or bone sometimes break free and float within the confines of the joint, diminishing joint mobility. The *synovial membrane*, a band of tissue that lines the joint capsule and secretes synovial fluid, can become irritated and inflamed, stimulating the membrane to produce more and thicker fluid. The extra fluid causes obvious swelling, called *effusion*, within the joint and can also create pain by stretching the joint capsule.

Osteoarthritis can occur in a single joint or in many joints simultaneously. Six joints in the foot and ankle are most commonly affected: the big toe joint (first metatarsophalangeal joint), the joint between the first metatarsal bone and the cuneiform bone behind it (first metatarsocuneiform), the joint between the ankle bone and the navicular bone in front of it (talonavicular), the joint between the heel bone and the cuboid bone in front of it (calcaneocuboid), the joint between the heel and ankle bones (subtalar), and the ankle joint (see also figures 1.1 and 1.2 in chapter 1). The incidence of osteoarthritis increases with age, which explains why it is commonly called "wear and tear" arthritis and degenerative joint disease.

As we age, the framework of protein within cartilage diminishes, leading to a gradual breakdown of the cartilage. This category of cartilage degeneration is termed *primary osteoarthritis*. There may be a genetic component to primary osteoarthritis, as it is not uncommon to see the condition appear in successive generations within the same family. Another category of the condition, *secondary osteoarthritis*, occurs as a result of an identifiable cause. Anything that increases the mechanical load on a joint or creates uneven pressure distribution across it can wear down or wear away the cartilage. For example, obesity, abnormal foot mechanics, repetitive stress in sports or exercise, bone deformity, joint instability, and muscle weakness all add to the strain on joints. Foot and ankle joints are particularly susceptible to wear because of the repetitive stresses they are exposed to daily. In addition, any event or condition that damages joint cartilage may initiate osteoarthritis. Examples include trauma, prior surgery, inflammatory arthritis, diabetes, infection, certain medications, and nutritional abnormalities.

Some people have osteoarthritis without symptoms, although a frequently used joint, such as those in the ankle, will most likely develop symptoms eventually. For other people, osteoarthritis can be severely painful and limiting. Pain can range from a dull ache to a sharp, burning sensation. Pain and stiffness are often present in the foot with the first few steps taken after resting, but they generally ease after ten to fifteen minutes of activity. However, the pain may be made worse by increasing the level of activity or by spending a long time on the feet. If you have osteoarthritis, you may find that your affected joints are particularly sore in humid or cold weather. The affected joint may not move as well as before, and sometimes the joint loses its ability to move altogether.

People with osteoarthritis sometimes have an altered gait such as a limp because of the pain and reduced or lost ability to move the joint. With movement, you may feel a grinding or grating sensation, known as crepitus, within the joint. If bone spurs are present around the joint, a callus may form. Swelling, redness, or warmth around the joint occur in some, but not all, cases of osteoarthritis. If your osteoarthritis is severe, you may experience cramping or spasms in muscles near the affected joint, as you overuse these muscles in an attempt to protect the painful joint.

In the physician's office, you may undergo various tests to confirm a diagnosis of osteoarthritis. Oftentimes, all that is needed is an x-ray to show the extent of arthritis, including narrowing of the joint space, whitening of the bone under the cartilage, bone spurs, loose bones, and cysts within the bones. A special x-ray called a computerized tomography (CT) scan, and magnetic resonance imaging (MRI) are additional tests that can be used to evaluate further the extent of arthritis and deformity within a joint. These tests are often done in preparation for surgery.

It's not always clear from symptoms and diagnostic imaging whether a joint is affected by osteoarthritis or by another type of arthritis. In this situation, the podiatrist may send you for blood work or may test the fluid found within the affected joint. Removing a sample of fluid requires a technique called aspiration, which is done under local anesthetic. Aspiration involves surgically puncturing a joint (*arthrocentesis*) with a needle and draining out some fluid into a syringe. In addition to providing a fluid sample, joint aspiration can relieve pressure, and therefore pain, by removing excess fluid. Joint aspiration can also be used to collect blood after a traumatic injury.

At present, no treatment can halt the deterioration of cartilage. Rather, the goal of treatment for osteoarthritis, and in fact for any type of arthritis, is to decrease the pain and swelling while improving your ability to function. A podiatrist tailors the treatment regimen to address the joints involved, depending on how severely they're affected. The first treatments to try are resting and modifying your activities, especially to avoid activities and shoes that increase stress on the painful joint. For example, if you have an arthritic big toe joint, avoid kneeling down to sit with your big toe forced into extension and don't wear high-heeled shoes. Supportive shoes, over-the-counter arch supports, and custom-made orthotics can relieve pain. They will also control the foot's position, as well as protect, support, and offload weight from the arthritic joint. If you have a rigid, severely arthritic joint, you may find a brace useful.

If you have osteoarthritis, you can continue to exercise, provided the activity is modified to minimize the intensity and frequency of stress placed on the painful joint. Instead of using a treadmill or step machine, which causes repetitive stress and impact to the foot and ankle, consider swimming, using an elliptical machine or stationary bike, or doing light weight training. Once the acute pain subsides within the arthritic joint, we encourage exercise, because it promotes joint mobility, discourages the joint from becoming stiff, and strengthens the muscles that support the foot joints. Exercise is also thought to stimulate cartilage growth and bone strength. Warming the joint and surrounding muscles with a heat pad, hot water bottle, or warm shower before exercising can help to reduce joint stiffness as you begin an activity. Similarly, applying ice after exercise helps to limit swelling and muscle spasms.

A variety of medications can be used to limit or control the symptoms of osteoarthritis. Nonsteroidal anti-inflammatory medications, such as ibuprofen, naproxen, or Relafen can be used for short-term pain relief, but the potential for negative side effects makes their long-term use inappropriate. Tylenol is often tried first because it has few side effects. It provides pain relief, but it has minimal anti-inflammatory effects. Note, however, that Tylenol is not recommended if you have liver disease and should be used under the care of a physician if you take blood thinners, such as coumadin. You can apply topical medications directly to the skin over and surrounding an arthritic joint. We recommend capsaicin cream, BENGAY or other menthol-based ointments, or Volataren gel, which is available only by prescription. Some over-the-counter supplements are thought to be beneficial as well, including omega fish oil, chondroitin sulfate and glucosamine, multivitamins, ginger, and calcium. Before you start taking any of these supplements, however, consult with your physician or at least with a pharmacist, because many over-the-counter and herbal supplements have side effects and drug interactions.

For an acutely painful joint, cortisone injections into the joint may provide significant short-term, and sometimes long-term, relief of pain and swelling. Synvisc is another injected medication used to treat osteoarthritis, more commonly for larger joints like the knee and hip than for foot and ankle arthritis. Synvisc provides a temporary improvement in joint cushioning and lubrication. If you have significant joint disease, you may be referred to a rheumatologist to help establish the most appropriate medication regimen.

Another nonsurgical treatment option is physical therapy, which focuses on strengthening the tendons and muscles surrounding the affected joint and increasing or maintaining its mobility, as well as relieving pain. When conservative measures fail to adequately relieve the pain, you might consider surgery. The goal of surgery is to provide pain relief with improved overall function of the foot and ankle. Surgical options for the foot and ankle depend on which joint is involved.

Overactive Immune System: Rheumatoid Arthritis

Rheumatoid arthritis is a progressive autoimmune disease, which means that the immune system is overactive so that the body mistakenly attacks its own tissues. It is a systemic condition that creates inflammation and tissue degeneration within multiple joints in the body. Other organ systems can also be involved; for example, the lining around the heart (pericardium) and the lining inside the lungs (pleura) may become inflamed. With a defective immune response, chemicals and enzymes are released into joints, and over time, they create inflammation and thickening of the synovial lining of joints, a condition called *synovitis*. As the synovial membrane thickens, it produces excess synovial fluid, which causes swelling in the affected joints. The chemicals and enzymes released by the immune system also damage cartilage, bone, tendons, capsules, and ligaments. As the disease progresses over the years, joints become unstable and may be destroyed or deformed, resulting in permanent disability.

Nobody knows, at present, what causes rheumatoid arthritis. There is strong evidence that genetics plays a role in the development of the disease, and some people believe there may be chemical or environmental influences as well. Other possible causes include bacterial, viral, and fungal infections. Smoking has also been linked as a possible contributing factor.

Rheumatoid arthritis occurs about three times more frequently in women than in men, and it generally becomes evident after age 40. The small joints of the body are often affected first, so early signs of the disease tend to appear in the foot. Usually, multiple joints are affected bilaterally, meaning that the same joints are affected on each side of the body. In the foot, the joints of the forefoot are most commonly involved, but any joint in the foot can develop rheumatoid arthritis.

Initially, the symptoms of rheumatoid arthritis can be mild, and you may be free of symptoms for long periods—weeks or even months—with no obvious signs of the disease in the arthritic joints. When the disease is "active," however, the symptoms can be unpleasant. They include joint stiffness that lasts for an hour or more after rest before the joints finally "loosen." The affected joint is often painful, red, warm, and swollen. Systemic signs that can accompany the localized joint symptoms when the disease is active include fatigue, loss of energy, loss of appetite, and muscle stiffness.

Other problems that can develop in the foot as rheumatoid arthritis progresses are posterior tibial tendonitis (chapter 5); hammertoes, bunions, and metatarsalgia (chapter 8); plantar fasciitis and Achilles tendonitis (chapter 9); and tarsal tunnel syndrome (chapter 10). Calluses or corns (chapter 6) can form over areas with bony outgrowths, along with the possibility of developing an underlying bursitis, or worse, an ulcer, in areas exposed to excess pressure. If rheumatoid arthritis targets the joints of the midfoot, then midfoot collapse (loss of the arch) often occurs, and when hindfoot joints are involved, a common problem is hindfoot eversion, or pronation (turning outward).

Rheumatoid arthritis may also create inflammation within blood vessels, referred to as *vasculitis*, which impedes blood flow to the extremities. Vasculitis can lead to skin fragility and thinning as well as the potential for poor healing. A typical sign of vasculitis in the lower legs and feet is the development of black lines, called *splinter hemorrhages*, underneath the toenail plates.

Another characteristic common with longstanding rheumatoid arthritis is the presence of nodules within the soft tissues of the foot (*rheumatoid nodule*). These rheumatoid nodules most often occur over areas with a bony prominence or in areas subjected to repetitive pressure. The nodules become painful if they come into contact with surrounding structures, and they may become ulcers with chronic, repetitive stress.

The diagnosis of rheumatoid arthritis is usually made by or with the assistance of a rheumatologist. In addition to having blood taken, you will likely undergo some tests to evaluate inflammation, look for markers that are specific to rheumatoid arthritis and other inflammatory arthritis, and assess any effects of the arthritis on other organs, such as the kidneys and liver. The physician may do a joint aspiration, as described in the section on osteoarthritis, as well as send you for x-rays and MRI. If you meet four of seven criteria, then you are diagnosed with rheumatoid arthritis. The criteria are morning stiffness for longer than one hour for at least six weeks in a row, arthritis and swelling in more than three joints for at least six weeks, arthritis of hand joints for at least six weeks, symmetrical arthritis for at least six weeks, the presence of subcutaneous nodules, a positive rheumatoid factor (determined from a blood test), and x-ray evidence of joint erosion.

Treatment of rheumatoid arthritis aims to alleviate symptoms of pain and inflammation, prevent further deformity and destruction of joints, and maintain your functional capacity. Initial medications to relieve pain and inflammation include Tylenol, aspirin, nonsteroidal anti-inflammatory drugs (NSAIDs), and oral or injected steroids. Physicians discourage the use of NSAIDs for longer than a few months because of the potential for gastrointestinal side effects such as abdominal pain, stomach ulcers, and bleeding. Newer NSAIDs, such as Celebrex, have fewer of these side effects and may be used for several months to years.

Steroids are more effective than NSAIDs in reducing acute symptoms, but they have the potential for significant side effects, including weight gain, skin thinning, facial swelling, weakened bones (osteoporosis), bruising, muscle wasting, and deterioration of larger joints. The use of oral steroids is typically reduced as symptoms improve. Steroids injected directly into the affected joint are very effective at decreasing pain and inflammation as well as improving joint function. However, any one joint can receive only a limited number of injections, because excess steroid can contribute to further joint damage.

Once the pain and inflammation are under control, other medications can be taken to halt progressive damage and deformity to joints. These medications attempt to suppress the immune system and limit the production of destructive enzymes within joints. Examples of these medications include methotrexate, gold salts, Plaquenil, Imuran, Remicade, and Enbrel.

Other treatment options are similar to those used for osteoarthritis. Omega-3 fish oil is thought to have anti-inflammatory effects. Topical menthol-based creams, such as BENGAY, capsaicin ointment, and prescription Voltaren gel, relieve discomfort. You may find it helpful to wear supportive and accommodative shoes, a custom-made orthotic, or a brace to protect and support affected joints as well as offload weight and pressure from them. We encourage you to continue with regular exercise to maintain joint mobility and to strengthen supporting muscles.

Consider surgery if the conservative treatments are inadequate. The goal of surgery is to eliminate pain and to assist in restoring use of the foot and ankle. As with osteoarthritis, surgical options for the foot and ankle depend on which joint is involved. The common foot problems that frequently occur in conjunction with rheumatoid arthritis, as noted earlier, are discussed along with treatment options in other chapters of this book.

Crystals in the Joints: Gout

Gout is an arthritis that occurs when the body has difficulty processing uric acid. Uric acid is a substance normally present in our bloodstream. Our bodies produce it during the metabolism of proteins called *purines*. Purines are formed naturally in the body, and we also consume them in the foods we eat. The body eliminates uric acid mainly via the kidneys, with a small percentage leaving through the gastrointestinal tract. With gout, the body either produces too much uric acid or, more commonly, has difficulty removing it. As a result, the blood contains too much uric acid (a condition called *hyperuricemia*), which crystallizes and gets deposited into joints, tendons, and the surrounding soft tissues. The immune system responds to the presence of uric acid in and around a joint by releasing inflammatory chemicals. This causes the joint to become red, hot, swollen, and painful. Gout is more common in men than in women.

The inability to appropriately metabolize purines is usually an inherited trait, but other factors contribute to the development of gout. Some of these factors are eating too many protein-rich foods; consuming alcohol; being obese; having kidney disease, cancer, diabetes, high blood pressure, hyperlipidemia (excess fats or lipids in the blood), or hypothyroidism (insufficiently active thyroid gland); or taking certain medications (aspirin, thiazide diuretics, niacin, antirejection medications used in organ transplants, chemotherapy). Gout also may be initiated by injury to a joint, dehydration, fever, or surgery.

The primary symptom in gouty arthritis is rapid onset of a red, hot, swollen, tender joint. The pain comes from the physical presence of crystals within the joint as well as from the significant inflammation within the surrounding soft tissues. Symptoms commonly begin in the middle of the night or first thing in the morning. The pain can be so severe that even the pressure of a bed sheet on the foot is unbearable. Typically, an attack of gout lasts no longer than ten days, and it often improves after a few days. These acute flares of inflammation may occur more frequently with time. Also, over time, gout may become more destructive of the body's tissues, causing cartilage and bone damage. Uric acid crystals can accumulate in the soft tissues, resulting in white, chalky soft tissue masses called *tophi*. These tophi can lead to complications including ulcers around the joint (although sometimes in soft tissues away from a joint), kidney stones, and a clogged filtering mechanism in the kidney, which causes kidney disease. Gout, and the subsequent development of tophi, usually targets areas of the body that are relatively cool and farthest from the heart, which explains the prevalence of gout in the foot and ankle.

If you go to a podiatrist with suspected gout, the physician may perform a joint aspiration, as described in the osteoarthritis section, to diagnose the

condition. You may also have blood drawn for various tests. A high level of
uric acid in the blood is not, on its own, sufficient to diagnose gout. A small
percentage of the general population has elevated uric acid levels and never
develops arthritis or kidney disease. On the other hand, some people who
experience an acute attack of gout have uric acid levels within normal limits.
Last, you may have x-rays taken to assess joints for damage, including the
erosion of surrounding bone and the presence of tophi.

The goal of treatment for acute gout is to relieve pain and inflammation
and to make walking more comfortable. Medications to try first are NSAIDs
such as ibuprofen or Naprosyn. The prescription indomethacin is a type of
NSAID that is very effective at easing the symptoms of acute gout. However,
if you have a history of kidney disease, liver disease, or gastrointestinal problems, then you must use caution with these medications and take them only
under the direction of a physician. Oral or injectable steroids are effective in
decreasing pain and inflammation and can be used safely even if you have a
history of kidney disease or gastrointestinal problems. Colchicine is another
useful prescription medication for dealing with an acute attack of gout. You
take it every hour until the pain and swelling resolve or until you experience
gastrointestinal side effects such as nausea or diarrhea. Other treatment options for acute gout include ice, elevation, and immobilization. Options for
immobilization range from using a stiff-soled shoe or surgical shoe, which
reduces the load on joints in the forefoot, to using a walking cast, which
stabilizes and reduces the load on joints in the front, middle, and back of the
foot as well as in the ankle.

For people with longstanding gout, there are several options for medications
to prevent recurrent attacks of arthritis, tophi formation, and kidney disease.
Allopurinol decreases uric acid production by inhibiting an enzyme that par-
ticipates in purine metabolism. Probenicid promotes the elimination of uric
acid by the kidneys. These two medications are not to be used during acute
flares of arthritis because they can actually increase the severity of the attack.

If you have gout, it is also important to examine your diet. *Avoid* the foods
listed in table 11.1, which increase the amount of uric acid in the blood, and
add the foods listed in table 11.2 to your diet, because they help to reduce
the amount of uric acid in the blood. Stay hydrated by drinking adequate

amounts of water—eight to twelve 8-ounce glasses of water a day. Drinking enough water is critical to help excrete excess uric acid and minimize the risk of gout.

Table 11.1: Foods that increase uric acid

Meats	Fish	Vegetables	Others
Liver	Anchovies	Asparagus	Alcohol
Poultry	Any fish	Cauliflower	Candy
>8 oz/day	>8 oz/day	Green peas	Dry beans (e.g.,
Red meat	Sardines	Mushrooms	red, white,
Smoked meats	Shellfish	Spinach	black, pinto,
			kidney)
			Jam/jelly
			Sugar sodas
			Syrup

Table 11.2: Foods that help to reduce uric acid

Fruits	Dairy products	Dietary supplements	Others
Blackberries	Cheese	Celery extract	Coffee
Blueberries	Milk	Chondroitin	Water
Cherries/		sulfate	
cherry juice		Vitamin B5	
Purple grapes		Vitamin C	
Raspberries			

Surgery is not a treatment option for gout but may be appropriate to treat any conditions or complications that develop as a result of having gout. For example, with tophi formation in chronic gout, the overlying soft tissues may ulcerate and become infected. Surgery may be necessary to drain the infection and remove the unhealthy ulcerated tissue and tophi.

Chapter 12

Tendon Injuries

WE'VE ALL HEARD OF tendonitis and of sports figures pulling or even rupturing a tendon, but it's hard to appreciate the discomfort—and often serious pain—unless it's happened to you. Unfortunately, tendon injuries are relatively common, especially in certain sports, although they are not limited to athletes and people who exercise. Tendon injuries rarely happen in an instant, unless a tendon is cut or badly stretched during a sudden traumatic event. Rather, they tend to occur over time, with age, with repetitive movements, with overuse. In this chapter, we briefly describe tendons and categories of tendon injury and then discuss causes, symptoms, and treatments of three tendon injuries: injuries to the peroneal tendon, injuries to the flexor hallucis longus tendon, and Achilles tendon rupture. Two other tendon injuries are described elsewhere in this book: posterior tibial tendonitis in chapter 5 and Achilles tendonitis in chapter 9.

Types of Tendon Injury

Tendons are relatively inelastic but flexible and strong bands of fibrous tissue that connect muscles to bones. Similar to rope, tendons consist of multiple interwoven fibers, called *collagen*, between which are threaded nerves and blood vessels. In areas where tendons wrap around bones or ligaments and where they lie adjacent to bone, most tendons are encased in a sheath. This sheath produces a fluid to reduce friction and allow the tendon to glide easily as it transmits the force of muscle contraction to bone. Tendons are designed to withstand tension, but if they are continually strained by a repetitive stress or they are exposed to a sudden violent stress, they may be injured. In addition to overuse, repetitive activities, and sudden exertion, tendons are susceptible to injury from infection, trauma, collagen vascular disease (an abnormality with the blood vessels that supply the collagen fibers), gout, rheumatoid arthritis, and increasing age. Tendons tend to have a relatively limited blood supply, which also increases their susceptibility to damage and injury.

Tendon injuries typically are classified into three categories: tenosynovitis, tendonitis, and tendinosis. *Tenosynovitis* occurs when the tendon sheath becomes inflamed, which restricts the movement and gliding of the tendon and causes pain. The tendon and its sheath may join together; an abnormal joining of two tissues like this is called an *adhesion*. *Tendonitis* refers to an acute injury with damage and inflammation of a tendon, causing swelling and warmth in the area surrounding the tendon as well as pain when using the tendon.

Tendinosis describes chronic damage to a tendon from continuous overuse. The damage occurs over a long period, with an accumulation of small tears to the collagen in and around the tendon. As a result of the degeneration, the tendon may become thinner, or thicker, and longer if fraying or tearing occurs within it. Unlike other tendon injuries, tendinosis doesn't involve inflammation. Athletes, manual workers, and other people who perform the same repetitive activities daily are more likely to develop tendinosis. The symptoms are stiffness and pain. The pain with tendinosis is often intermittent and can occur immediately after rest, because small fibers of scar tissue that began to form during rest are torn upon walking. Pain can also occur with mild or moderate activity, depending on the amount of tendon involved and the severity of the tendinosis.

With both tendonitis and tendinosis, the tendon tries to repair itself with the help of cells called *fibroblasts*, which are woven amongst the collagen fibers along with the blood vessels and nerves. The scar tissue that forms where the tendon repairs itself is inherently weaker than the original tendon tissue, placing the tendon at risk for further tearing and failure. Complete rupture of a tendon is extremely rare, but it can happen when a tendon has become severely degenerated or when a tendon is subject to violent trauma or laceration (large-scale tearing).

Peroneal Tendon Injuries

The lower leg has two peroneal tendons, which, along with the muscles they attach to, are called the *peroneus brevis* and *peroneus longus*. The tendons begin on the outer side of the lower leg and travel behind the outside of the ankle-bone, where they lie in a cartilage-covered groove and are held in place by a strong ligament called the *peroneal retinaculum*. From here, the peroneus brevis continues along the outer part of the hindfoot and inserts into the midfoot. The peroneus brevis assists in lifting the foot out and up. The peroneus longus follows the peroneus brevis to the midfoot and then continues horizontally under the foot to insert into the inside of the arch. The peroneus longus helps to stabilize the arch. Where the tendons run along the outer heel bone, a small piece of bone, the *peroneal tubercle*, sticks out, and the tendons run above and below it. The peroneal tubercle is a normal part of the anatomy, but in some people, it is larger than usual and can be a source of tendon irritation.

The peroneal tendons are most frequently damaged behind and below the outside of the anklebone. This location has relatively few blood vessels, and the tendons may rub directly against the bone as they change direction before traveling into the foot. Injury to the ligament that holds the tendons in place can also allow them to partially slip out of the groove behind the ankle. The point where the peroneus brevis inserts into the midfoot is another common location for peroneal tendon injury. This injury usually occurs in individuals with an inherited foot structure where the base of the fifth metatarsal is prominent on the outside of the midfoot. A metatarsus adductus (inward rotation of the forefoot relative to the hindfoot) also creates an abnormally prominent fifth metatarsal base (shown in figure 4.6 in chapter 4).

The causes of peroneal tendon injury are numerous. With aging, tendons lose their already limited elasticity and become more susceptible to injury. Certain foot types and positions, such as a high-arched foot and the outward position of a flat foot (chapter 5), as well as a foot with restricted upward movement at the ankle, can add strain to the peroneal tendons. High-top shoes and boots and footwear that tends to fit poorly, such as ice skates, can press directly on the tendon and contribute to its injury. Loose outer ankle ligaments that create an unstable ankle increase the chance of spraining an ankle and tearing the peroneal retinaculum ligament. Repetitive ankle motion from walking, running, and being on the feet all day, especially in jobs that require repeated actions like climbing, pushing, pulling, and squatting, leads to wear and tear on the tendon. Inflammatory arthritis causes tendon inflammation as part of the disease process, and the deformed joint or associated bone spurs can also rub on, degrade, and inflame surrounding tendons. In some people, the groove that the peroneal tendons lie in behind the anklebone is flat or convex, and in other people, an extra tendon or a low-lying muscle occupies space in the groove. In either of these cases, the peroneal tendons are displaced from the groove, and they may rub against the outside anklebone, which is not covered with smooth cartilage, and become injured.

The symptoms of peroneal tendon injury usually occur along the outside of the ankle and can include any combination of pain, swelling, warmth, stiffness, and a snapping feeling. There may be pain with use of the tendon, or pain and stiffness after rest. With tendinosis, there may be accompanying weakness in the tendon that makes it difficult to move the foot up and out, or the foot may remain in an inverted position as stronger tendons overpower the weakened peroneal tendons.

A podiatrist can usually diagnose a peroneal tendon injury with only a physical examination of the ankle and foot. He or she will press in the area of the tendons over the outer portion of the ankle, which usually elicits pain. It's usually also painful to move the foot upward and outward, which you try first on your own and then with the physician pressing against the foot to prevent it from moving. Another indicator of injury is when the tendons have been displaced from the groove behind the outer ankle, which a podiatrist can see by moving the ankle through its range of motion. If necessary, x-rays can be taken to identify bone injury and ankle instability, and an MRI can evaluate the extent and location of the tendon injury, as well as associated bone and soft tissue injuries. Ultrasound can also be used to evaluate the tendons. If tendon weakness is detected, the podiatrist may recommend that you have nerve conduction studies and electromyography to determine if a nerve entrapment syndrome is also present (chapter 10).

Treatment of peroneal tendon injuries is designed to control and improve symptoms and to restore function. Initial treatment for any tendon injury is a combination of rest, elevation, ice, and nonsteroidal anti-inflammatory medications. Immobilization protects the foot and ankle and allows the tendon to heal. This treatment can range from a removable ankle brace for milder cases to a hard cast on the lower leg for cases of significant tendinosis. If these treatments are successful in addressing the symptoms, then we recommend that you continue treatment with physical therapy to improve balance, stability, and strength. Wearing a custom-made orthotic is helpful to address an abnormal foot position that could lead to the tendon injury recurring.

Surgery is reserved for nonresponsive cases. The type of surgical repair and reconstruction depends on the extent to which the tendon and tendon sheath are damaged and the extent to which the surrounding soft tissue structures and bone are involved. With tenosynovitis, the inflamed synovial tissue is removed and any necessary bone procedures are done. Surgery for tendonitis and tendinosis depends on the extent of damage and may consist of removing portions of damaged tendon and repairing the tendons and surrounding ligaments. Sometimes synthetic grafts or tendon grafts from elsewhere in the foot are used to augment the damaged tendon. In people with a convex groove and displaced tendons, the outer anklebone can be ground down to deepen the groove. If you also have a high-arched foot or another foot position that contributed to the tendon injury, the surgery may be able to address it at the same time.

Whether with conservative treatment or surgery, it can take from weeks to months for a tendon injury to heal. After surgery, you will have a below-knee cast or a CAM walker, and you must stay off the foot for four to six weeks. After this, you move to protected weight bearing in a walking cast for an additional two to four weeks, and then return to wearing supportive shoes, ideally in combination with a custom-made orthotic or a lace-up ankle brace. Most people wear an ankle brace for an additional three to six months, although we recommend that athletes continue to wear the brace when participating in their sport. A tendon injury may recur, but you can minimize the chances by using an orthotic or brace. With tendonitis and tendinosis, the tendons are usually slightly weaker after repair, but not noticeably. With complete tendon rupture and repair, you may have noticeable weakness.

Dancer's Tendonitis: Injuries to the Flexor Hallucis Longus

Dancer's tendonitis refers to an injury that commonly occurs in dancers, particularly ballet dancers, though other people get this injury, too. The injury (which may be tenosynovitis or tendinosis, not only tendonitis) is to the *flexor hallucis longus* tendon. This tendon is in the lower leg and helps to move the foot downward (plantarflexion) to assist in stabilizing the ankle. It also bends the big toe down to provide it with strength during push-off in the gait cycle. The tendon attaches to a muscle, called the flexor hallucis longus muscle, which runs down the back of the lower leg. The tendon begins behind the ankle and travels through three tunnels made of fibrous tissue and bone on its way to the big toe.

The tunnels correspond to the areas where the tendon is most commonly injured. The first tunnel is directly behind the anklebone (talus), where two bony protrusions, referred to as tubercles, confine the tendon, and a ligament holds it in place. The second tunnel is on the inside of the heel bone (the tarsal tunnel; see chapter 10), where the tendon travels underneath another tubercle. The third channel is located underneath the big toe joint, where the tendon lies beneath and between the two small bones called sesamoids. The tendon then inserts into the end of the big toe.

Flexor hallucis tendon injury is classified into the three categories described earlier: tenosynovitis (also known as checkrein deformity), tendonitis, and tendinosis. Injury to the flexor hallucis tendon tends to occur in active people. It is especially common in ballet dancers who use the *en pointe* position, which can stretch the tendon beyond its physiological limits. Sports such as running, football, soccer, and tennis that require repetitive pushing off from the front of the foot can also injure the tendon. Other contributing factors include an inherited low-lying muscle that takes up space within one of the tunnels that the tendon lies in, possibly forcing the tendon out of its normal location within the tunnel and creating tendon irritation, and the presence of a soft tissue mass that presses on the tendon. Trauma to the tendon itself or to surrounding bony structures can also result in tendon dysfunction. People with extremely flat feet (hyperpronation), diabetes, and rheumatoid arthritis are all at greater risk of developing problems with the flexor hallucis tendon.

Symptoms include ankle pain, both at the back and on the inside of the ankle, as well as swelling. You may experience tingling in the arch of the foot, and it may be painful to bend the ankle or the big toe. Often the big toe has a diminished range of motion, and when you try to extend it, the toe may snap or trigger. Typically, activity exacerbates the pain, and rest relieves it.

A podiatrist will do a physical examination and may order x-rays or an MRI to diagnose an injury to the flexor hallucis longus tendon. X-rays are used to identify the presence of a fracture, tumor, or an *os trigonum* (see the box in this chapter). If the patient is a ballet dancer, the physician may ask for an x-ray while the dancer stands in the *en pointe* position. MRI evaluates the tendon and its sheath, as well as any associated soft tissue masses.

Treatment of an injured flexor hallucis longus tendon is initially with rest, nonsteroidal anti-inflammatory medications, and gentle stretching exercises to stimulate increased blood flow to the injured tendon. One stretching exercise involves sitting on a bed with legs outstretched and only your heels hanging

An Extra Bone: Os Trigonum Syndrome

The os trigonum is a small bone at the back of the ankle that occurs in only a small proportion (less than 15 percent) of the population. The flexor hallucis longus tendon travels directly adjacent to it. Os trigonum syndrome occurs with inflammation of ligaments surrounding the bone, of fibrous tissue connecting the os trigonum to the anklebone, or of the ankle joint itself. It is commonly seen in people who participate in activities requiring repetitive downward motion (plantarflexion) of the ankle, which can squeeze the os trigonum between the ankle and heel bones. Symptoms of os trigonum syndrome are pain and swelling at the back of the ankle. The syndrome is treated in the same way as tendon injuries, with rest, ice, and possibly immobilization. Nonsteroid anti-inflammatory medications and cortisone injections can also be used. Surgery to remove the bone may be considered if conservative treatments do not resolve the symptoms. Os trigonum syndrome can occur at the same time as or separately from an injury to the flexor hallucis longus tendon.

over the edge. In this position, push your foot down to point the toes and then extend your big toe upward, holding this position for five seconds. Do three repetitions two or three times a day. In addition, the stretching exercise recommended for plantar fasciitis can also be helpful (see the "Achilles Tendon and Plantar Fascia Stretches" box in chapter 9). Custom-made orthotics and ankle braces or straps can relieve irritation of an inflamed sheath. It is also wise to stop wearing any badly worn-down shoes and, for dancers, to refrain from dancing on hard surfaces. (Once the tendon has healed, a ballet dancer can go back to using the *en pointe* position.) You may find it beneficial to go to physical therapy for massage or ultrasound treatments. Steroid injections are usually avoided for fear of further weakening the tendon. If the injury is underneath the big toe, the toe can be strapped to limit strain on the tendon. If these conservative treatments aren't successful, you should stop all physical activities and immobilize the foot for four to six weeks.

Consider surgery if the conservative treatments don't relieve symptoms. Surgery involves removing areas of damaged tendon and repairing the tendon where possible, releasing adhesions within the tendon sheath and removing any soft tissue or bony structures, including the os trigonum, that impede the tendon as it lies in the tunnels between the ankle and big toe. After surgery, you will have a fiberglass below-knee cast or a CAM walker and must stay off the foot for four to six weeks before moving to protected weight bearing in a walking cast for an additional two to four weeks. Wearing an orthotic can also be helpful when first returning to regular shoes. Dancers and athletes may find it helpful to wear a brace when they initially return to their dance or sport after significant surgery to repair or reconstruct the tendon. Once a tendon has been injured, it is more susceptible to future injury. Wearing an orthotic or brace can help prevent the chance of recurrence.

Achilles Tendon Rupture

The Achilles tendon is a large, strong, ropelike cord that connects the muscles in the calf to the back of the heel bone (calcaneus). When we contract the calf muscles, the Achilles tendon bends the ankle to move the foot downward (plantarflexion), giving us the ability to rise up on our toes and to run, jump, and climb. An area of the Achilles tendon about 4 to 6 centimeters (1 to 2 ½ inches) above its insertion into the heel bone has a particularly low blood supply and is therefore the most common site for tendon damage and rupture. When it ruptures, the tendon either partially or completely tears. A partial tear means that some of the tendon fibers have torn while others haven't, like a rope unraveling and leaving a few strands intact.

The chance of rupturing the Achilles tendon increases with age, because tendons lose their limited elasticity with use. People with diabetes or rheumatoid arthritis also have a greater incidence of Achilles tendon rupture. Some medications increase the risk as well, including corticosteroids and fluoroquinolone antibiotics (e.g., ciprofloxacin, Avelox). People with tight or weak calf muscles, whether inherited or acquired, and people with a previous Achilles tendon injury are also more prone. Most frequently, however, the Achilles tendon ruptures in people participating in sports. Athletes are at greatest risk if they abruptly change their training or if their sport necessitates sudden bursts of jumping, pivoting, or running. Although the unconditioned athlete or "weekend warrior" is particularly at risk, Achilles tendon rupture can happen to well-conditioned and elite athletes, too. The actual rupture of the tendon is caused by a sudden and forceful downward (plantarflexion) or upward (dorsiflexion) movement of the foot or by direct trauma.

If your Achilles tendon ruptures, you will feel, and possibly hear, a pop at the back of the ankle. It may feel like you were kicked or hit with a baseball bat in the back of the ankle. The area suddenly feels severely painful, and it swells and bruises. It's actually possible to feel a gap or soft spot at the site of the rupture. Even with the tendon ruptured, you may be able to walk, bend the ankle, and move the foot downward, because other tendons that assist with foot plantarflexion remain intact. However, you will find it impossible to rise up onto your toes with an Achilles rupture. Most people are able to walk with a limp after a rupture, although walking is not advisable. If you suspect that you've ruptured the Achilles tendon, get medical attention quickly. Surgical repair is best done within a day or two of the injury to avoid having to use tendon transfers or grafts.

A podiatrist diagnoses an Achilles tendon rupture with a physical exam. One common test is for you to lie on your stomach while the physician squeezes your calf muscle. With an intact Achilles tendon, your foot should move downward, but if the tendon is ruptured, your foot won't move at all. X-rays show any accompanying bone injury, such as a heel bone fracture at the tendon's insertion point or bone spur formation at the back of the heel bone. If there is any question about the location or extent of the tear, you may be sent for MRI.

The recommended treatment for an Achilles tendon rupture depends on your activity level. Elite athletes and very active people usually move straight to surgical repair, which involves sewing, or suturing, the tendon back together. After surgery, you must keep off the foot for four to six weeks and gradually move to protected weight bearing in a walking cast for an additional two to four weeks. For people who are less active, conservative care can be tried as a first option. In this case, the foot is immobilized and you stay off it for six weeks, followed by an additional two to four weeks of protected walking.

Whether you have surgery or undergo conservative care with immobilization alone, you may be able to begin physical therapy during the two to four weeks of protected walking. Physical therapy will strengthen and stretch the tendon, increase the ankle's range of motion, and re-educate the proprioreception mechanism that gives you a sense of where your foot and ankle are. Proprioreceptors relay the foot's position to the brain, but rupturing the Achilles tendon can delay or diminish the signals traveling along these nerve pathways. Most comparison studies show that a surgically repaired tendon and a conservatively managed tendon have a similar result when it comes to the function and strength of the Achilles tendon. The only difference is a higher likelihood of re-rupturing the tendon in people who underwent immobilization rather than surgery.

If an Achilles tendon rupture is not treated or is inadequately treated, there are consequences. The person walks with an *apropulsive gait*, which means that the foot can't effectively push off during the toe-off stage of walking. Rising up on the toes will be difficult, if not impossible. Also, the toes may contract over time into hammertoes, because the toe flexors substitute for the loss of the Achilles tendon by firing longer and harder than normal.

Part Three
People with Special Foot Needs

Chapter 13

Foot Problems that Start
in Childhood

WE ALL WANT OUR children to be healthy and to grow and develop without having to endure health problems that require repeated visits to doctors, clinics, and hospitals. Inevitably, we don't all get what we want. Any childhood illness or health problem is stressful, both for the child and for the parents and other family members. Fortunately, most foot and ankle problems in children can be treated so that as a child continues to grow, the feet function normally and without pain. Although treatment is usually successful, it's important to take a child to a physician and seek treatment as soon as possible, because some foot and ankle conditions have long-term complications. In this chapter, we discuss some of the more common childhood foot problems, how they occur, and how they can be treated. Some of the conditions that begin in childhood become problematic later, in adulthood, so we discuss treatment of adults in this chapter, too.

Feet Turned Inward: In-toeing

When a child's feet turn inward as he or she walks or runs, the foot position is termed *in-toeing*, also known as pigeon toed. Most cases of in-toeing—as well as cases of out-toeing, the opposite foot position (discussed below)—are thought to be simply a variation of normal development that will correct spontaneously as a child grows. A child may have both feet turned in (or out), or only one foot. There are three main causes of in-toeing: metatarsus adductus (a C-shaped foot), tibial torsion (twisting of the lower leg bone, the tibia), and femoral rotation (inward positioning of the thigh bone, the femur).

Metatarsus Adductus

Usually noted at birth, *metatarsus adductus* is a foot position in which only the front half of the foot turns inward. The foot has a C shape, with a concave inner border and a convex outer border, as shown in figure 13.1. A metatarsus adductus foot may be flexible, where the foot can be straightened manually; semi-rigid, where the foot can be only partially straightened manually; or rigid, where the foot cannot be straightened manually. Metatarsus adductus is a common birth condition, occurring in 1 of every 1,000 births and equally between boys and girls. The left foot tends to be more frequently affected because of fetal position within the uterus. Sometimes, a child with metatarsus adductus also has hip dysplasia (abnormal structure of the hip).

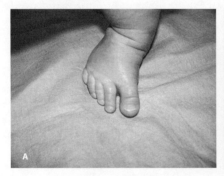 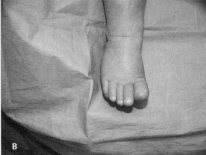

Figure 13.1. Metatarsus adductus is a C-shaped foot. This child had a cast on the foot and leg for several months to correct the deformity.

Causes of metatarsus adductus include the baby's position in the uterus, a family history of the deformity, the position an infant sleeps in (lying on the stomach with the feet turned inward), and abnormal muscle position or muscle tightness in the foot. A podiatrist diagnoses the condition with a physical examination of the child's foot and possibly with x-rays to evaluate its severity and the position of the bones in the foot. It's fairly common for other foot and lower leg problems to occur at the same time as metatarsus adductus, including tibial torsion and femoral rotation, described below, and a flat foot, discussed in chapter 5.

What the doctor aims to accomplish in treating metatarsus adductus is to create a straight and functional foot. Treatment depends on the child's age and medical history, the severity of the condition, and the flexibility of the foot. A flexible metatarsus adductus responds well to daily stretching and manipulation, which is performed by pressing on the inside of the foot at the big toe joint while keeping the heel vertical and applying counter-pressure on the outside of the midfoot and heel. A child should also avoid sleeping on his or her stomach. For a more rigid metatarsus adductus, we usually recommend putting a cast on the foot and lower leg. Casts are most effective with infants between the ages of three and eight months. The cast is removed and reapplied every one to two weeks for a duration of six to twelve weeks. The purpose of a cast is to gradually reduce the inward bend of the forefoot while simultaneously holding the heel straight to avoid creating a deformity in the back of the foot. Foot braces and special shoes used to be the primary treatment for rigid metatarsus adductus, but these devices have fallen out of favor because if they're not used properly, they can cause other foot problems, such as skin irritation, a broken-down arch, or a valgus hindfoot. However, some physicians still recommend using a brace after casting to maintain a correct foot position.

After the cast comes off, the child can wear a modified oxford shoe made from a straight last with an open toe and high top, as shown in figure 13.2. A pad is applied to the shoe on the inside of the first metatarsal and a counter-pressure pad is applied to the outside of the shoe over the cuboid bone. An arch pad and a wedge on the inside of the heel are also used in an attempt to maintain the correction and to protect the arch from being broken down.

If your child's metatarsus adductus has not responded to conservative therapy, you might consider surgical treatment. However, surgery should not be done until a child is at least two years old. If your child needs a surgical procedure to correct metatarsus adductus, ask about the surgeon's experience with these cases. The surgery should be done only by specialist surgeons who perform these procedures frequently. The appropriate surgical procedure depends on your child's age, the severity of the deformity, and any other conditions that are also present, such as tibial torsion or femoral rotation.

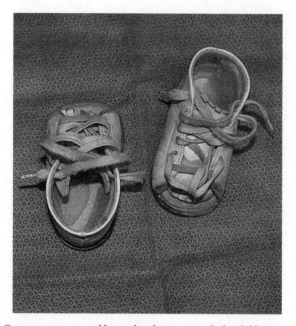

Figure 13.2. Once a metatarsus adductus has been corrected, the child wears a straight last, high-top, open oxford shoe with felt pads inside it to preserve the arch and maintain the correction.

Surgery in a child younger than six years old usually involves releasing the soft tissues around any tight muscles or ligaments in the midfoot. In an older child, the surgery usually involves the bones as well. Procedures can include making cuts to the metatarsal bones in the forefoot or the cuneiform and cuboid bones in the midfoot with isolated or combination procedures. These may include removing triangular wedges of bone or using triangular bone grafts to help straighten the foot. After either soft tissue release or a bone cut procedure, the child wears a cast for six to twelve weeks and must not put any weight on the corrected foot. When the cast is removed, the child wears a protective boot for an additional two to four weeks to gradually put weight on the foot. Finally, the child wears a supportive shoe and custom-made orthotic. A metatarsus adductus sometimes recurs when the child begins to walk, but it is usually relatively minor and can be treated with in-shoe modifications and stretching.

Some parents try reversing a child's shoes—putting the left shoe on the right foot and vice versa—in an attempt to correct a metatarsus adductus. This is *not* a good idea, because the dramatic and sudden change may break down the arch and cause an additional deformity.

Internal Tibial Torsion

The lower leg has two bones, the fibula and the tibia. Sometimes, the tibia is twisted inward, called *internal tibial torsion*. At birth, the tibia has no twist to it. After birth, the tibia gradually twists outward to create a straight lower leg. On occasion, however, the outward twist doesn't progress as it should, and both the leg and the foot remain turned inward. Most often, parents first notice the in-toe appearance of their child's foot when he or she begins to walk. The child may seem to be very bowlegged. A podiatrist will examine your child's foot and leg to evaluate the range of motion in the joints; whether the tibia or the femur, or both, are twisted; and whether there's a difference in the length of the legs. The podiatrist will ask whether there is any family history of vitamin D deficiency or bone metabolic disorders. The child will also have a complete neurological examination, because altered limb rotation occurs with some neuromuscular diseases, such as cerebral palsy and spina bifida.

Most internal tibial torsion conditions resolve on their own by the time a child is 4 to 6 years old. A few never resolve, but most children with such a condition function perfectly well and don't have any limitations or changes to the foot in compensation for the tibial torsion. In-toeing shouldn't affect your child's ability to walk, run, play, or function normally. If your child's condition is severe, he or she may trip more, especially when running, because the swing foot hits the stance leg. In the rare situation when the internal tibial torsion remains at ages 6 to 8 years and the child is in pain and can't function normally, bone cuts can be made in the tibia to make the leg rotate outward.

Internal Femoral Rotation

At birth, the thighbone, called the femur, is rotated inward while the hip joint is rotated outward. As a child grows during the first few years, the femur usually rotates outward and the hip joint inward to create a straight upper limb. If this process is altered by trauma, hip dysplasia, loose ligaments, or weak muscles, the thigh will turn inward, creating an inward appearance to the entire limb referred to as *internal femoral rotation,* or *anteversion.* This rotation is slightly different from the tibial torsion described above in that the bone itself is not twisted (torsion); rather, the position of the femur is rotated. Children with internal femoral rotation have kneecaps that point toward each other. These children also often sit on their knees with the lower legs underneath them and with their feet turned inward (a W position, or reverse tailor's position).

As with internal tibial torsion, a podiatrist diagnoses internal femoral rotation by physically examining the child (see above). Most children with this condition do not require treatment, because the condition resolves on its own by the time the child is 6 to 8 years old. If your child is diagnosed with internal femoral rotation, he or she will likely function normally and without any physical limitations, even during the first 6 to 8 years, while the condition is resolving. We encourage children with this condition to participate in activities that require external rotation of the hip, such as riding a tricycle; skating, including in-line skating; and ballet. Also, you and other caregivers should discourage your child from sitting in a W position and encourage him or her to sit in the tailor's position (cross-legged) instead. In the rare cases of severe deformity, with pain in the hip or knee, particularly with a kneecap that doesn't glide correctly when the knee moves (called poor patellar tracking), you might consider surgery to cut and rotate the femur bone.

Feet Turned Outward: Out-toeing

When a child's feet turn outward as he or she walks or runs, the foot position is termed *out-toeing*. Out-toeing occurs when either the tibia or the femur twist outward or when normal inward rotation of the hip is delayed. Out-toeing is much less common than in-toeing. When it does occur, you will probably notice the condition within the first two years of your child's life. Out-toeing most often resolves on its own within the first year after a child begins to walk. Braces and special shoes are rarely helpful. If out-toeing causes pain, problems with the foot's function, or poor patellar tracking, as described above, then you might consider surgical realignment. The surgical procedures would be the same as those described for correcting internal tibial torsion and internal femoral rotation.

On Tiptoes: Toe Walking

The Achilles tendon—the strongest tendon in the body—is an extension of the three calf muscles: the two heads of the gastrocnemius and the soleus. It begins just below these muscles and continues along the back of the lower leg to insert into the back of the heel bone. When the Achilles tendon contracts, it plantarflexes the foot, or makes the foot move downward, as in pointing the toes. If the tendon or the calf muscles, together called the *Achilles complex*, are too tight, the foot stays in a downward position, with limited ability to bend the ankle and bring the foot back up. This foot position is called *equinus*. Severe tightness in the Achilles complex makes a person walk on tiptoes.

In a child, there are three main reasons for toe walking: idiopathic (cause unknown) toe walking, called Prancer's syndrome, shown in figure 13.3; toe walking due to spasticity; and toe walking due to a paralytic muscle disease. Other causes of toe walking, more common in adults than children, are trauma to the ankle, a bone spur that creates a blockage in the ankle, a cast that keeps the ankle in a downward position for a prolonged period, and high-heeled shoes worn regularly. Regardless of the cause of toe walking, over time the foot tends to compensate for the lack of upward motion at the ankle by moving up and out into a pronated position. This pronation of the foot may create a flat foot, which causes additional problems (see chapter 5). The body may also compensate for a tight heel cord in other ways, including hyperextending the knee; taking the heel off the ground early when walking (which produces an identifiable bopping gait); and developing *lumbar lordosis* (curvature to a part of the vertebral column so that the buttocks point excessively backward).

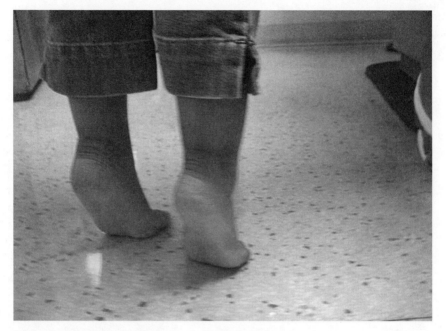

Figure 13.3. A child walks on the toes in Prancer's syndrome.

Idiopathic toe walking occurs either because a child walks on the toes out of habit or because a child is born with a short Achilles tendon, which is a nonspastic congenital condition. (Congenital means the condition happens during fetal development but is not genetic, or inherited. It may be due to fetal position in the uterus, development variation, or other reasons.) You will first notice obvious toe walking when your child begins to walk. Idiopathic toe walking occurs symmetrically in both limbs; if only one limb is affected, the cause is not idiopathic. If prompted, a child with idiopathic toe walking is usually able to get his or her heel down to the floor. The child has normal tendon reflexes, balance, and coordination, and initially, the range of motion in the Achilles complex and the ankle may be within normal limits. However, habitual toe walking can lead to the Achilles tendon becoming permanently contracted, with the ankle in a fixed downward position.

Toe walking from spasticity means that the nerves supplying the calf muscles tend to fire too much or too frequently, making tendon reflexes overactive. Spasticity commonly occurs with neuromuscular diseases such as cerebral palsy, stroke, and spinal cord tumors. A toe walker with a neuromuscular disease will have a toe-to-toe gait, rather than the normal heel-to-toe gait, and the child will not be able to touch his or her heel to the ground. The onset of toe walking may be gradual when spasticity is the cause, and the toe walking may occur in either both legs or only one leg.

Toe walking from certain paralytic muscle diseases, such as muscular dystrophy, occurs because of weakening in the muscles at the front of the leg that bring the foot toward the shin. In this case, the calf muscles and Achilles tendon overpower these weak muscles, creating a downward position in the foot and causing toe walking. Paralytic muscle diseases can also weaken the calf muscles by replacing the normal muscle tissue with scar tissue, leading to muscle and tendon tightening. Someone who toe walks due to paralytic muscle disease often has decreased tendon reflexes. The child may or may not be able to touch his or her heel to the ground, depending on the extent of the disease. The onset of toe walking may be gradual, and the toe walking may occur in either both legs or only one leg.

If your child is a toe walker, a podiatrist will watch as he or she walks and will do a physical examination. The physician tests the calf muscles and the Achilles tendon for strength and range of motion to assess which component is tight. This assessment is done by having your child lie on his or her back or sit upright with legs straight out in front. The physician moves the ankle through its range of motion with the knee straight and then a second time with the knee bent. This test is called a Silverskiold test. The podiatrist may also have x-rays taken of the foot and ankle to determine if bone spurs at the front of the ankle are limiting ankle motion. If the podiatrist suspects that your child's toe walking is caused by a neuromuscular disease, then a referral will be made to a neurologist, who may do nerve conduction tests to find out which nerves could be involved (see chapter 10). A neurologist may also request x-rays or an MRI of the spine to look for lesions that may be causing a nerve entrapment syndrome.

If the diagnosis is idiopathic toe walking that has developed from habit, and if the physical examination is normal, then your child will simply be monitored with follow-up appointments every few months. If the physical examination suggests tightness in the Achilles complex, then stretching exercises, physical therapy, and splints can all be used to stretch the Achilles tendon. If your child is young and has congenital shortening of the Achilles tendon, a series of casts on the lower limb can be used to gradually stretch the tendon. The cast is changed weekly for six to twelve weeks. The correction may be maintained with an ankle–foot orthotic until the skeleton matures. The goal of this orthotic is to prevent the problem from either progressing or recurring and to prevent the foot from compensating into a pronated posi- tion. As long as there's no pain, your child will still be able to walk, run, and play sports while wearing the orthotic. If the problem does not respond to this conservative treatment, surgery can be done to lengthen either the entire Achilles tendon or just the gastrocnemius portion of the tendon.

If you have a young child who toe walks because of muscle spasticity, treatment involves serial casting followed by maintenance with an ankle–foot orthotic until skeletal maturity. If this treatment doesn't work, surgical options include lengthening the tendon or injecting a small amount of botulinum toxin, widely known as Botox, into the calf to weaken the spastic muscles. The side effects of Botox injection are minimal and include temporary pain and bruising at the injection site, greater than desired muscle weakness, and temporary adjustment to walking with the weakened muscles. If your child toe walks because of a paralytic muscle disease, he or she will be treated by stretching the Achilles tendon and splinting and bracing the foot and ankle. Where there is scarring and contraction of the muscles, we don't advise sur- gical lengthening, because this will further weaken the tendon complex.

An Extra Midfoot Bone: Accessory Navicular Syndrome

Some children are born with an extra piece of bone or cartilage next to the navicular bone on the inside of the midfoot. The bone tends to protrude from the foot on the inside of the arch. This extra bone is called an *accessory navicular*, and sometimes an *os tibiale externum*. It is completely surrounded by the posterior tibial tendon as the tendon inserts into the navicular bone. In some children, the accessory navicular doesn't create a problem, and in oth- ers, it leads to a debilitating and painful syndrome. *Accessory navicular syndrome* is common in children with flat feet. It usually occurs in both feet.

The syndrome can be initiated by trauma, irritation from shoes rub- bing against the prominent bone, and overuse of the posterior tibial tendon. Symptoms include pain, redness, and swelling on the inside of the foot. A child may feel pain when rising up onto the toes or when wearing certain shoes. The symptoms usually first occur in adolescence as the bones are developing, but sometimes they begin in adulthood. The signs that a podiatrist looks for in diagnosing accessory navicular syndrome include a prominent bone on the inside of the foot and discomfort when testing the strength of the posterior tibial tendon. The tendon's strength can be tested by asking the patient to rise up onto the toes or to push his or her foot toward the body's midline while the podiatrist uses a hand to resist the movement. X-rays will show the accessory bone, and an MRI may be ordered, more commonly in an adult than in a child, to evaluate the posterior tibial tendon for injury.

Initial treatment of accessory navicular syndrome consists of rest, ice, compression with an ACE bandage or soft cast, and nonsteroidal anti-inflammatory medications. If symptoms are severe, a podiatrist may recommend immobilization for four to six weeks with either a weight-bearing or non-weight-bearing cast. If your child responds well to these treatments, we recommend that he or she use a custom-made orthotic to provide continued support to the foot (see chapter 16). If your child's symptoms don't improve with conservative treatment, there are surgical options.

Surgery usually involves removing the accessory navicular bone, cutting away a portion of the posterior tibial tendon and reattaching it to either the navicular bone or the cuneiform bone to maintain tension on the tendon, and smoothing out any outgrowth on the navicular bone itself. Recovery includes wearing a cast and keeping weight off the foot for six weeks followed by a gradual return to walking in a protective boot for two to four weeks. After this time, your child wears supportive shoes with a custom-made orthotic, which we recommend that he or she use for life when doing a lot of physical activity. Physical therapy may be necessary to strengthen the tendon, provide pain relief, and increase the foot's range of motion.

Bone Connections: Tarsal Coalition

Bones that are normally separated by a joint are sometimes connected to each other by cartilage, fibrous tissue, or bone. When such a bone connection occurs in the foot, it is usually between the tarsal bones, which include the talus, calcaneus, cuboid, navicular, and cuneiforms (see chapter 1), hence the name *tarsal coalition*. A tarsal coalition is a congenital condition that can occur in either one foot or both feet. Depending on the location of the tarsal coalition, movement of the hindfoot can be significantly limited, leading to adaptive changes in the foot. For example, to compensate for loss of motion in the hindfoot, the midfoot often comes up and out into a pronated position, which results in a flat foot. When a person with a tarsal coalition rests or sits, the foot might stay fixed in a pronated position.

Symptoms can begin in childhood, usually as the bones mature in adolescence, but can be delayed until adulthood. Symptoms are sometimes initiated by trauma, such as an ankle sprain. The tarsal coalition causes symptoms of pain on the top of the midfoot, in the hindfoot, and toward the front of the outer ankle when walking or standing. Pain is often worse with activity and when walking on uneven terrain, and it is relieved with rest. Other symptoms are tiredness in the legs and muscle spasms in the foot or leg. The child may have a rigid flat foot and may walk with a limp because the subtalar joint is unable to compensate for or adapt to changes in the terrain. There may also be stiffness in the foot with limited ability to move the foot inward or outward.

A podiatrist diagnoses a tarsal coalition with a physical examination and imaging, such as x-ray, MRI, or CT scan. Initial treatment is designed to diminish the pain and limit motion and stress across the affected joint. Treatment options include immobilization, nonsteroidal anti-inflammatory medication, cortisone injections into the painful area, strappings for support and to limit pronation, and custom-made orthotics. If conservative therapy fails to relieve the discomfort, you might consider surgery. If your child is young and active and has no arthritis, then he or she can have the tarsal coalition removed so that the bones are no longer joined. After the surgery, the foot is immobilized for four to six weeks, followed by aggressive physical therapy to maximize the range of motion in the affected joint. Finally, the child returns to wearing supportive shoes and may need a custom-made orthotic. For an adult patient who also has joint arthritis, surgical fusion to connect the bones in the affected joint is usually recommended. This procedure is followed by immobilization in a cast for ten to twelve weeks with gradual return to weight bearing in a protective walking cast.

Bone Degeneration: Osteochondrosis

In a growing child, the bones lengthen as new cells are produced by an area of cartilage in a bone called the *growth plate*. If blood supply to the growth plate of an individual bone is interrupted in a child, a portion of the bone dies, defective bone forms at the growth plate, and later, bone regrows at the site. This phenomenon, for which the exact cause is unknown, results in a condition called *osteochondrosis*. Possible reasons include rapid growth, trauma, heredity, vascular (blood vessel) injury, overuse or repetitive stress, abnormal weight and pressure on the bone, or dietary imbalance.

A diagnosis is made with a physical examination and imaging, such as x-ray, bone scan, and MRI. X-rays, if taken early in the process, may be normal, but as the disease progresses, the bone appears white and fragmented. Bone scans show decreased blood flow to the affected bone, while MRI may be used to differentiate osteochondrosis from other conditions. Osteochondrosis can occur with any bone in the body, but we discuss only the two most common sites in the foot, at the navicular bone (Kohler disease) and at the metatarsal head (Freiberg infraction).

Kohler Disease

Osteochondrosis of the navicular bone is called Kohler disease. It usually develops between the ages of 2 and 9, and it occurs more frequently in boys than in girls. The child often limps and feels tenderness or pain on the inside of the arch. This area may also have localized swelling, warmth, and redness. Treatment is aimed at reducing the pain and inflammation. The majority of children with Kohler disease recover fully with conservative treatment, and surgery is rarely needed. Conservative treatment is nonsteroidal anti-inflammatory medication and immobilization in a weight-bearing or non-weight-bearing cast. Once the symptoms resolve, we recommend that your child use a custom-made orthotic. An x-ray of the bone will appear normal within six months to four years of the condition resolving, and the bone will grow normally.

Freiberg Infraction

Osteochondrosis of the metatarsal head, most commonly the second or third metatarsal head, is called Freiberg infraction. Girls are affected more frequently than boys. Some children have no symptoms, while for other children, the condition is extremely painful. Possible causes include a short first metatarsal, a long second metatarsal, repetitive mechanical overload (for example, from jumping on the toes), or wearing high-heeled shoes, which force an excess load onto the forefoot. A child with Freiberg infraction experiences pain in the front of the foot, and the pain is made worse with increased activity. The child may also walk with a limp. Pain and swelling are centered over the metatarsal head and the joint where the toe meets the foot (metatarsophalangeal joint), and there may be pain when moving the toe as well.

Early diagnosis and treatment of Freiberg infraction is critical for minimizing damage to both the bones and the joints involved. As the disease progresses, there may be significant damage to the cartilage in the joint with collapse of the metatarsal bone. Loose pieces of bone can also appear in the joint, and bone spurs can form at the edges of the joint. Treatment is targeted at reducing pain and increasing joint function. If diagnosed when the disease first appears, your child's foot should be immobilized in a weight-bearing or non-weight-bearing cast until all symptoms are gone. In more advanced cases, when bone destruction has occurred, treatment includes modifying the shoes to minimize pressure on the area, wearing shoes with rocker soles to take weight off the front of the foot, using pads to relieve pressure, and if your child is older and the growth plate has closed, injecting cortisone into the joint.

If your child's symptoms are not relieved with conservative treatment, there are numerous surgical options, all of which have had successful outcomes. The best procedure to use depends on your child's age, how active he or she is, the degree to which the bone and joint are involved, and how damaged the bone and joint are. When damage is minimal, the surgery attempts to preserve the normal anatomy of the foot using a joint salvage procedure. Joint salvage procedures include cutting out spurs in the joint, making cuts to the metatarsal bone to shorten it and decompress the joint, bone grafting of the affected metatarsal head to stimulate bone healing, or elevating healthy cartilage from the bottom of the metatarsal head upward to replace the damaged cartilage. When the joint has been severely damaged, joint-destructive procedures are recommended. Joint-destructive options include removing a portion of the head of the metatarsal, replacing the joint with an implant, or fusing the joint. The course and length of recovery from surgery depends on the procedure performed.

Pain in a Growing Heel: Sever Disease

The heel bone (calcaneus) in a growing child develops in two areas, one in the main body of the bone and a smaller one at the back of the heel. Between these two areas is the growth plate, or *apophysis*, a section of cartilage that assists in producing bone cells for growth. At around 14 to 16 years of age, the cartilage disappears, and the back section fuses with the main body of the heel bone. Sometimes, the growth plate becomes inflamed, resulting in a condition called Sever disease, or *calcaneal apophysitis*. This disease typically occurs in children between the ages of 10 and 14 years, when they're going through a growth spurt. As a child grows, the bones elongate first, and muscle growth lags behind, causing tightness in the muscles. In Sever disease, the heel bone's growth plate, located where the Achilles tendon inserts into the heel bone, experiences increased tension from the Achilles tendon and becomes inflamed and painful.

The most common causes of Sever disease are overuse of the Achilles tendon, commonly from sports like soccer, football, and running, and repetitive pulling of the Achilles tendon on the growth plate. Tight calf muscles, flat feet (overpronation), and sport shoes such as soccer cleats are known contributing factors. Symptoms are chiefly mild swelling around the heel and pain at the back or sides of the heel, as well as discomfort during or after physical activity. Sever disease is often self-limiting: once the growth plate closes, the condition ends. However, children experiencing Sever disease are frequently in a lot of pain, which limits the activities they participate in, so we recommend that children be assessed and treated by a podiatrist.

Treatment is aimed at both reducing the symptoms and alleviating the pull of the Achilles tendon. Heel lifts placed in the shoe, calf stretching, ice, and wearing supportive, cushioned shoes are helpful. We often recommend reducing the length of time a child with Sever disease plays a sport. We don't advise removing your child from an activity unless the condition does not respond to initial treatment. If pain continues, a podiatrist may recommend that the child take a nonsteroidal anti-inflammatory medication such as Children's Motrin or an analgesic such as Tylenol. A period of immobilization may be necessary for unresponsive cases. Once the symptoms resolve, custom-made orthotics can help to prevent recurrence of the problem.

Short Metatarsal Bones: Brachymetatarsia

When one of the five metatarsal bones is too short, the condition is called *brachymetatarsia*. The fourth metatarsal and toe are affected most frequently, but it can occur in any one of the metatarsals. It is usually diagnosed in an infant and occurs in girls more than in boys, most often affecting both feet. Brachymetatarsia results when the growth plate in the metatarsal closes prematurely, causing the bone to be significantly shorter than it should be. With a shortened metatarsal, the pressure and load distribution in the front of the foot is altered. Excess weight is now transferred to the adjacent bone or bones, often resulting in pain and frequently the formation of a callus beneath these bones (see metatarsalgia in chapter 8). In addition to the bone deformity, the surrounding soft tissues also shorten or contract. These tissues include the flexor and extensor tendons to the toe as well as the joint capsule and ligaments of the joint between the toe and the metatarsal. The toe itself becomes short, elevated, floppy, and relatively nonfunctioning. If the toe is elevated above the other toes, shoes rub and press on it, causing pain and callus formation. In addition to the physical discomfort, young women, in particular, can be affected emotionally and psychologically by the appearance of their feet.

Most cases of brachymetatarsia are either congenital (developing in the uterus without a genetic link) or inherited (having a genetic link). Other possible causes include trauma, postsurgical change, Down syndrome, Apert syndrome, Albright osteodystrophy, sickle cell anemia, dwarfism, and poliomyelitis. Conservative treatment includes the use of pads or cushions to protect the affected toe from pressure. Open-toe or extra-depth shoes are also helpful in alleviating pressure from an elevated toe. Over-the-counter insoles with padding or custom-made orthotics can be used to relieve pressure under the affected areas at the front of the foot. If nonsurgical options fail to provide adequate pain relief, surgical reconstruction is worth considering. Surgical options include lengthening the shortened metatarsal, shortening the adjacent metatarsals, and correcting the position of the shortened toe. Recovery time following surgery depends on the procedure.

Overlapping and Underlapping Toes

Not everyone's toes lie perfectly straight, but in some people, one or more toes overlap or underlap the adjacent toe. Both overlapping and underlapping toes are thought to be congenital conditions. The position of the baby in the uterus contributes to overlapping.

Overlapping toes, usually present at birth, are common among children. The fifth toe (the "baby" toe) is most frequently affected, followed by the second toe (the toe next to the big toe). The affected toe is positioned up and rotated inward. The skin on the inside of the toe is tight, as is the tendon that brings the toe up (extensor tendon). Sometimes, but not always, the toe dislocates from the joint where it meets the foot. An overlapping toe is usually free of pain in a child, but it may cause symptoms of pain, bursitis, and callus formation in an adult. Children rarely outgrow overlapping toes, so the toe or toes should be treated in childhood.

Treatment in a young child or infant involves stretching and taping the affected toe into a corrected position for at least six to twelve weeks. Surgery can be considered for children who don't respond to conservative treatment and for adults who have a very painful deformity. In a child, surgery can consist of skin lengthening on top of the toe, skin tightening on the bottom of the toe, tendon release or transfer, joint release, and pinning of the toe in a corrected position. In an adult, this procedure may be recommended with the addition of bone procedures to remove a portion of a toe bone (arthroplasty) or permanent stiffening of the toe (arthrodesis; see chapter 8). Recovery typically entails walking in a surgical shoe for six weeks with a gradual return to normal shoes. Elderly people who are not good surgical candidates can benefit from conservative treatments that aim to relieve pressure on the toe by using pads, modifying shoes, or wearing extra-depth shoes, or in rare cases, where reconstruction is inappropriate, amputation.

Underlapping toes, known medically as *clinodactyly* and commonly as curly toes, is thought to be a congenital condition, but the cause is unclear. Figure 13.4 shows a child's foot with a curly toe and other toe conditions. There may be a muscular imbalance in which the tendon that flexes (brings down) the toe is firing longer and harder than the tendon that extends (brings up) the toe. The third, fourth, and fifth toes tend to be the ones to underlap. An underlapping toe assumes a downward and inward position, so that the toe goes beneath the adjacent toe. A painful callus often forms on the outside of the toe or outside the nail plate. The pain is made worse by wearing tight shoes and by spending a long time on the feet.

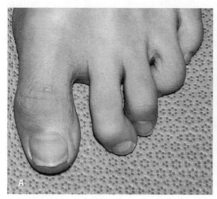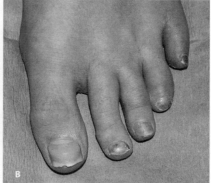

Figure 13.4. (A) This child has two flexible mallet toes (second and third toes), curly toe (fourth toe), and adducto-varus deformity (fifth toe). (B) The toes were corrected with a soft tissue procedure to snip the tendon and joint capsule on the bottom of the toes.

An underlapping toe that does not press or only mildly presses against the adjacent toe may not need treatment. When treatment is suggested for an infant, it initially entails taping or splinting the toe into a straight position (this is rarely successful in children over 6 months of age), and the parent is instructed to manually stretch the toe. Conservative treatment in adults involves applying pads or cushions and avoiding tight shoes. A podiatrist can routinely cut away the callus to relieve symptoms. If conservative care has been unsuccessful in a child or an adult, surgery is an option. The surgery aims to make the toe straight and involves cutting the flexor tendon; removing portions of the skin, tendon, and joint capsule to help correct soft tissues; and removing bone, if necessary. Recovery after this procedure takes four to six weeks with protected weight bearing in a stiff-soled surgical shoe and then a gradual return to normal shoes.

Choosing Shoes for Children

Teensy shoes may look cute on a baby, but babies don't need shoes and, in fact, should not wear shoes until they begin to walk. Wearing shoes too soon has the potential of putting unwarranted pressure on the foot. Soft socks or unrestrictive booties are safe for nonwalking babies. Once a child begins to walk, he or she is ready to wear shoes, but they should not be too heavy or have a very stiff or "sticky" sole, because this may make it difficult for the child to walk without tripping or falling down. The most important factor in choosing shoes for your child is that the shoes fit the feet properly. Never force a foot to fit. A properly fitting shoe should have a straight or normal last, a rounded toe box, an absorbent insole, and a strong, stable heel counter. It should also be flexible across the ball of the foot, such as a sneaker or runner. There should be a half-thumb's width (of an adult's thumb) between the longest toe and the end of the shoe. A child's shoe size can change as often as every three months, so check the fit of your child's shoes frequently and have his or her foot measured before fitting new shoes. Always check your child's feet for the formation of blisters or calluses, which indicate that shoes are not fitting properly.

Second-hand shoes are commonly used for children and, in general, are not a good idea unless the shoes were infrequently worn and are in good shape. As with shoes worn by anybody, whether adult or child, they lose their support and cushioning with wear. In addition, shoes become worn down in some areas because of a foot's shape or position when walking. A second child is unlikely to have exactly the same foot type and gait as the first. For example, if the first child wore down a shoe on the inside edges of the heel and sole, then the next child to wear the shoes would have his or her feet thrown to the inside edges of the shoe as well, regardless of the child's own foot position.

Chapter 14

Common Sports Injuries and the Sports Enthusiast's Foot

MANY PEOPLE PARTICIPATE IN some form of sport or exercise, some as elite athletes and many more for the pleasure of the sport and the associated health benefits. Sports and exercise injuries are common among both groups. The feet, ankle, and lower leg receive a large proportion of these injuries, because so many sports involve running or jumping or pushing on the feet. When people think of sports injuries, they often think of accidental injuries, but overuse injuries are perhaps more common. In either case, an injury can be acute and resolve with treatment or can become a chronic problem for the individual.

This chapter focuses on the causes, symptoms, and treatment of common foot and ankle injuries, but it is by no means inclusive of all possible injuries. Addressing all possibilities would take an entire book. Some injuries that occur frequently with certain sports are covered in other chapters of this book, such as the formation of blisters and calluses (chapter 6), metatarsalgia and predislocation syndrome (metatarsophalangeal capsulitis; chapter 8), and tendon injuries—which include posterior tibial tendonitis (chapter 5); Achilles tendonitis (chapter 9); and peroneal tendon injury, flexor hallucis longus tendon injury, and Achilles tendon rupture (chapter 12).

Injuries to the Sesamoid Bones

Beneath the head of the metatarsal that joins to the big toe are two small oval-shaped bones called the sesamoids. The sesamoids are an integral part of the big toe joint. They have two primary functions: to act as a shock absorber and to act as a fulcrum for the flexor tendon, which pulls the big toe downward. In effect, these bones are part of a pulley system that increases the force with which the flexor tendon pulls the big toe down as a person walks. This pulling down on the toe gives greater power with toe off in the gait cycle. The sesamoids are encased in a fibrous web of tendons and ligaments that hold them in place and stabilize the big toe. The top of the two bones is covered with cartilage to allow for smooth, pain-free motion where they join the big toe joint.

The sesamoid bones can sustain two different types of injury: *sesamoiditis* and *sesamoid fracture*. Sesamoiditis occurs when there is chronic inflammation of the sesamoids themselves, their surrounding soft tissue, and the connection point between them and the first metatarsal head. This condition usually results from repetitive, abnormal stress to the forefoot and specifically to the big toe joint. People who are prone to developing sesamoiditis are those who wear high-heeled shoes every day, those with a high-arched foot, and those who participate in sports and other activities requiring repetitive pushing off and jumping. Ballet dancers are particularly at risk, as are runners, sprinters, gymnasts, and people who play sports like basketball, tennis, soccer, and football. Sesamoid fracture occurs when repeated stress to the bones causes either a stress fracture—one or more hairline cracks on the surface of a bone—or a traumatic fracture, with complete breaking of the bone. Stress fractures can result from the same activities that cause sesamoiditis. Traumatic fracture may occur after hyperflexion or hyperextension of the big toe joint, or after a person falls from a height.

Both sesamoiditis and sesamoid fracture produce pain under the big toe joint. The pain worsens with activity and when the big toe is bent or straightened. With either injury, the range of motion in the big toe may be decreased. Sometimes, sesamoid injuries cause bruising on the ball of the foot.

Diagnosing the exact problem with sesamoids can be tricky, but it's critical to visit a podiatrist and have a correct diagnosis made. The sesamoids have a relatively poor blood supply, so delayed or inappropriate treatment risks cutting off the blood supply altogether, resulting in bone death, or *avascular necrosis*. This condition is extremely difficult to treat. If you go to a podiatrist with a suspected sesamoid injury, you will have x-rays taken to look for a bone fracture. Most likely, both feet will be x-rayed, even though the injury is typically only in one foot. In some people, the sesamoids naturally form in two separate pieces instead of one (referred to as a *bipartite sesamoid*), which is a normal anatomical variation, shown in figure 14.1, that may occur in as much as one-third of the population. Comparing an x-ray of the two feet helps to differentiate a bipartite sesamoid from a fractured sesamoid, because a bipartite sesamoid is usually present in both feet. In addition, a bipartite sesamoid has smooth, rounded edges whereas a fractured sesamoid may have jagged, irregular edges. If the podiatrist remains uncertain after examining x-rays, you may be sent to have a nuclear bone scan or MRI.

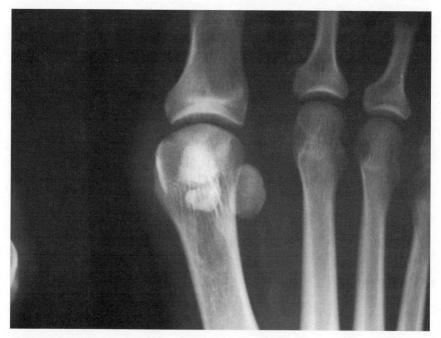

Figure 14.1. A bipartite sesamoid is a normal anatomical variation that some people are born with.

The treatment differs depending on the injury. Treatment of sesamoiditis includes taking nonsteroidal anti-inflammatory medication; limiting or ceasing the activity that caused the problem; padding the ball of the foot to offload pressure from the bottom of the big toe joint; wearing soft cushioned shoes with a low heel, rocker sole shoes, or a stiff plate in the insole; splinting the big toe into a downward position; and using custom orthotics. Stubborn cases may also benefit from steroid injections into the tissue surrounding the sesamoids. Once the acute symptoms resolve, exercises for the big toe help to strengthen the muscles and tendons and increase the toe's range of motion.

Treatment of a sesamoid fracture usually consists of some form of immobilization. For example, the big toe may be held with a splint so that it can't extend upward (dorsiflex), the ball of the foot may be padded, or you may wear a cast or CAM walker on the foot and ankle. We recommend aggressive treatment of a sesamoid fracture to avoid the risk of avascular necrosis, because treating avascular necrosis requires several months of immobilization and staying off the affected foot. Bone growth stimulation may be recommended to assist in healing both a sesamoid fracture and avascular necrosis.

If you have either sesamoiditis or sesamoid fracture that doesn't improve after ten to twelve weeks of treatment, you might consider surgery. Surgery for sesamoiditis and nonhealing sesamoid fractures usually consists of removing the affected sesamoid and repairing the surrounding soft tissues. Occasionally, an individual with a sesamoid fractured into two parts will have only the smaller fragment removed, but this technique risks a recurrence of the initial problem. Both sesamoid bones are not typically removed because this will alter and weaken the pulley mechanism of the flexor tendons and over time may cause contraction of the big toe (similar to a hammertoe). Some elite athletes have had a fractured sesamoid surgically repaired using screws and bone grafting, but the results are extremely variable. After sesamoid surgery, whether it was removed or repaired, most people are able to return to activities and sports without any problems.

A Sprained Big Toe: Turf Toe

If you sprain any component surrounding the big toe, or first metatarso-phalangeal joint, you have a condition called *turf toe*. Turf toe includes injury to the joint capsule, ligaments, sesamoids, big toe, or first metatarsal head. It commonly occurs after sudden hyperextension (upward movement) of the big toe, forcing the toe to extend beyond its physiological limits. Less commonly, turf toe is caused by sudden hyperflexion (downward movement) of the big toe. Turf toe is so named because this injury occurs frequently in athletes who play sports on artificial turf. Synthetic grass surfaces have a greater coefficient of friction than natural grass, meaning that the surface is more resistant to a foot sliding over it. Therefore, a player's foot can more easily become fixed against the ground and be injured. Despite the name, however, turf toe is not a condition isolated to activities on artificial turf. Any activity that requires a sudden push-off on a hard surface or a sudden stop that jams the toe against the shoe or that places the foot at risk of forceful extension will increase the chance of turf toe injury. In addition, the increasing demand for speed in athletes has altered shoe design to maximize flexibility in the forefoot at the expense of shoe stability. These shoes make forefoot injury more likely. Another cause of turf toe is wearing shoes that are worn out, because worn shoes become more flexible and place the foot at risk of forefoot injuries.

Turf toe injuries vary in severity and are graded accordingly. A grade 1 injury consists of minor stretching of the joint capsule and ligaments. Symptoms include soreness in the big toe joint with minimal swelling and no associated bruising. A grade 2 injury occurs with partial tearing of the joint capsule and ligaments. Symptoms are more diffuse pain spreading into the ball of the foot behind the big toe with moderate swelling and bruising. A grade 3 injury involves complete tearing of the joint capsule and ligaments, with possible associated damage to the sesamoids and first metatarsal head. Symptoms are extreme pain that is difficult to pinpoint along with swelling, bruising, and pain when trying to move the joint. X-rays are usually the only diagnostic tool required, although occasionally an MRI is necessary to further evaluate the joint.

The severity of the injury dictates the appropriate treatment. Fortunately, most turf toe injuries can be successfully treated without surgery. Initial treatment, regardless of the grade of injury, should be applying ice, elevating the foot, and resting the foot. As soon as the pain lessens, you should start moving the toe joint. When acute symptoms have diminished, a grade 1 injured toe can be taped or splinted. Grade 2 injuries may require a few weeks of immobilization and no weight bearing with a gradual return to walking in a protective shoe or boot. Athletes with a grade 2 turf toe may be able to return to their sport more quickly by inserting a thin carbon fiber insole into the shoe to prevent big toe dorsiflexion (upward movement).

Grade 3 injuries require two to six weeks of immobilization in a walking cast. These injuries also need to be evaluated for fractured or dislocated sesamoids and for a fractured big toe joint. (A fractured big toe joint involves a fracture of either of the two bones where they meet at the joint. The fracture can be at the base of the proximal big toe phalanx or at the first metatarsal head.) Any of these situations may require urgent surgical attention. Athletes recovering from a grade 3 turf toe should return to play only when they are able to change direction and run without pain.

Surgery may be necessary to treat bone and ligament injuries in an acute grade 3 injury and at a later time to treat problems that result from the initial turf toe injury, including persistent weakness in the toe and pain in the joint, chronic joint synovitis (inflammation of the membrane surrounding the joint), and arthritis.

Pain When Running: Shin Splints

Running and jogging, especially on hard surfaces like concrete, put the lower limb, ankle, and foot under a lot of stress. Frequently, the muscular attachments and connective tissue in front of the shinbone (tibia) are injured, resulting in a condition called shin splints. Shin splints tend to occur in runners and joggers who train improperly (inadequate stretching or warm-up period, or doing too much too soon), run on slanted surfaces (uphill, downhill, or a side-to-side slant from an overpronated foot position), or wear worn-down or inappropriate running shoes. Other factors that make a person more prone to developing shin splints are having a flat foot, an externally rotated hip (out-toeing; see chapter 13), or an internally twisted tibia (internal tibial torsion; see chapter 13). Typically, the symptoms of shin splints begin gradually with general pain at the front of the lower leg during the first few minutes of running. The pain usually eases as you continue to run in the early stages of shin splints. As the condition progresses, the pain becomes persistent with running, and the duration and intensity of pain worsens.

There are two types of shin splints, anterior and posterior, each with different causes and symptoms. Anterior shin splints produce tenderness along the front of the tibia about 5 to 10 centimeters above the ankle, which is where the anterior tibial muscle belly originates off the tibia. In people who have a tight heel cord (Achilles tendon), the anterior tibial tendon and the muscle it connects to must work harder and longer to lift the foot clear of the ground in the gait cycle. They also work longer to decelerate the foot as it hits the ground when a person runs downhill. In addition, if this anterior muscle and tendon are weak, either congenitally or from injury, they are less able to control the progression of the foot from heel strike to total foot contact (see chapter 1), so the foot tends to slap against the ground. When the foot repetitively goes through a rapid and forceful downward movement, as it does with running or jogging, microscopic tears occur within the anterior tibial muscle and at the point where the muscle attaches to the bone.

Posterior shin splints cause tenderness along the inner portion of the lower leg, which corresponds to the posterior ridge of the tibia. These symptoms commonly develop in a person with an excessively flat foot (see chapter 5), because the muscles on the inner leg are overworked as they attempt to maintain proper foot alignment. Over time, the strained muscles become inflamed.

Treatment for shin splints starts with decreasing the frequency and intensity of running or jogging. It's okay to continue exercising, but go easy on yourself. Ice can be applied after participating in an activity, and nonsteroidal anti-inflammatory medication may be used to ease tenderness or pain. Once the pain has diminished, treatment focuses on strengthening the lower leg and ankle muscles, as well as improving balance and coordination of the ankle. Full recovery can take up to six weeks, during which time you can maintain stamina by swimming or biking. Return to pre-injury activity levels should be gradual. Custom-made orthotics can help stabilize the foot and reduce the degree of pronation of a flat foot, thereby alleviating the abnormal strain on muscles. When first returning to a running sport, you may find that an ankle brace provides additional support until the symptoms completely resolve.

Rolled Over: Ankle Sprains

An ankle sprain happens when the ligaments that support the ankle are injured by a sudden force or twisting action. The ligaments can be stretched, partially torn, or completely torn (ruptured). There are several categories of ankle sprain depending on which ligament is injured. An outer ankle, or lateral, sprain is the most common, while high ankle sprains and inner ankle (medial) sprains occur much less frequently. A high ankle sprain involves a ligament between the two lower leg bones.

Given the wide range of motion in a normal ankle, you can appreciate that the ankle is a complex structure. It includes three bones: the anklebone (talus) and the two lower leg bones, the tibia and the fibula (shown in figure 1.3 in chapter 1). Ligaments, joint capsule, and tendons run across the ankle joint to hold everything in place. Ligaments connect one bone to another, hold tendons in place, and help to stabilize joints. There are ligaments at the front and back and on the inside and outside of the ankle joint. A ligament also connects the tibia to the fibula, a connection referred to as the *syndesmosis*.

A person typically sprains an ankle by rapidly twisting the foot either inward or outward to a point that exceeds the physiological limits of the joint capsule and ligaments. An inward twist, or inversion, means that the sole of the foot faces the midline of the body and your weight shifts over the outside of the ankle, causing a lateral ankle sprain. An outward twist, or eversion, means the sole of the foot faces away from the midline and your weight shifts onto the inner ankle, resulting in a medial ankle sprain. There is an increased risk of suffering a high ankle sprain while participating in contact sports. This injury involves the syndesmotic ligaments and occurs when one player falls on the back of another player's ankle while the foot is everted (turned outward). Predisposing factors for ankle sprains include poor muscle tone, a

high-arched foot, ankle instability, poor athletic conditioning, traumatic accident, obesity, and poor balance or coordination.

Some people hear an audible pop or snap when they initially sprain their
ankle. The injury causes swelling and pain around the affected structures, and
moving the ankle is often extremely painful. Bruising occurs over the injured
ligaments and may extend as far down as the toes. Most people are able to
walk—or at least hobble—on a sprained ankle, although it may be painful. If
you can't walk on the ankle, you may have broken a bone (although many
people can still walk with a fractured ankle).

A podiatrist will examine a sprained ankle to find out if you also injured
any other ankle structures, such as the tendons, the fifth metatarsal, the os
trigonum bone (see chapter 12), the cartilage, or the back of the heel bone
(calcaneus). You may have an x-ray done if the podiatrist suspects injury to a
bone or another joint in the foot. MRI is usually necessary only if you experience chronic pain after an ankle sprain. Immediate treatment for an ankle
sprain includes rest, ice, elevation, nonsteroidal anti-inflammatory medications, and possibly the use of an ankle brace or ACE bandage to control
swelling. Once an ankle sprain is diagnosed, a podiatrist may encourage you
to gently move the ankle and foot as soon as you can tolerate it in an effort
to help reduce swelling and to minimize the potential for scar tissue within
the joint (called *joint fibrosis*).

The goal of longer term treatment, especially for an athlete, is to restore strength, flexibility, and endurance to the pre-injury level. However,
it is equally important to reduce the chance of re-injury, which is common
following an ankle sprain because of lingering mechanical and functional
instability of the ankle. Mechanical instability means that structures like the
ligaments have healed in a lengthened fashion, and the ankle may be less stable
than it was prior to injury, referred to as *lateral ankle instability*. This instability makes an individual more susceptible to re-injury or recurrent sprains
when playing sports or walking on uneven ground. Functional instability
is harder to pinpoint. It involves proprioception, how the brain receives
nerve signals to sense the position of the body—or, in this case, the ankle and
foot. Proprioceptors tell the brain what position the foot is in at all times,
but an ankle sprain can interrupt these nerve pathways. Thus, after an ankle

injury, the automatic sense-of-position signals may be delayed or diminished, making it more difficult for the body to resist future ankle sprains. The goal of rehabilitation treatment after an ankle sprain, therefore, is to reduce the risk of both mechanical and functional instability by establishing a program of muscle strengthening and balance training. In addition to a podiatrist, you may have appointments with other professionals such as a certified athletic trainer or a physical therapist when recovering from an ankle sprain injury.

Hairline Cracks: Stress Fractures

Repeated stress on a bone can result in a hairline crack called a *stress fracture*. A stress fracture can be either an *insufficiency fracture*, where a bone is deficient and unable to bear a normal weight, or a *fatigue fracture,* where a normal bone receives an abnormal stress. Bone is a living tissue and is very adaptable. It can remodel itself—a process of removing old bone and forming new bone—to adapt and strengthen in response to external strains and stresses. However, bone needs time to remodel, so stress needs to be applied gradually. If a bone is put under excessive stress or if a bone has a deficiency in its remodeling capability, a stress fracture will occur. The most frequent sites for stress fracture in the lower limb are the tibia (one of the lower leg bones), the metatarsals in the forefoot, the calcaneus (heel bone), and the navicular (one of the midfoot bones).

People at risk of sustaining a stress fracture include runners and other athletes who run or play a sport on a hard surface, unconditioned athletes, and athletes and military trainees who overtrain or train improperly (improper stretching or warm-up, or rapid increase in the intensity, distance, or time of exercise). Ballet dancers are particularly susceptible to stress fractures of the sesamoids and second metatarsal head, while runners and other athletes tend most frequently to sustain tibial stress fractures. Other factors that contribute to stress fractures are aging; wearing inadequate shoes that are not sport-specific; having a high-arched foot, flat foot, bunions, or abnormal foot mechanics; having a nutritional or metabolic deficiency or a hormonal deficiency; having osteoporosis; or having peripheral neuropathy (nerve degeneration that can lead to muscle weakness, pain, numbness, or loss of balance and proprioception). In addition, prepubescent girls and women with menstrual irregularities are prone to stress fractures because of altered levels of the hormones estrogen and progesterone. These hormones affect bone mass and bone formation and predispose women to osteoporosis and decreased bone density.

An athlete who develops a stress fracture often recalls a concurrent change in the intensity, frequency, or duration of exercise, which may have taken place over several days or in a single event. Sometimes, the change is in the training surface or the type of shoes the athlete wears. The pain of a stress fracture frequently begins gradually as a dull ache at the end of a period of exercise. The intensity of the pain progressively increases over several days to the point that running cannot be tolerated. A few days of rest often relieves the pain only for it to return if the exercise is resumed. The location of the pain may be difficult to pinpoint and depends on which bone has the stress fracture. Metatarsal stress fractures often produce pain that spreads out over the top of the forefoot, while navicular stress fractures tend to cause vague discomfort on the top of the midfoot or the inside of the arch. In tibial stress fractures, the pain is often localized to the site of fracture on the tibia and can be similar to the pain of shin splints and exertional compartment syndrome (see the box in this chapter). A calcaneal stress fracture usually produces pain surrounding the back and bottom of the heel. Swelling, warmth, and redness often occur over the site of a stress fracture, but there is no visible bruising.

If you go to a podiatrist with a possible stress fracture, you will have an x-ray, although x-rays often don't show a stress fracture initially, because the fracture is literally only a hairline. Repeat x-rays taken two or three weeks later usually show the fracture, if it is truly present, because bone remodeling becomes more evident on the x-ray film, and a bone callus, which is part of the normal healing process, becomes visible. If a physical examination and your history suggest a fracture, then treatment should be started immediately, even if the first set of x-rays are negative. Other imaging tests are also available, including bone scanning, MRI, and CT scanning. Both bone scans and MRI will pick up a stress fracture, even early on, and CT scan is useful to evaluate one that is slow to heal or won't heal. A special scan, called a DEXA scan, may be ordered if the podiatrist suspects that you have

Compartment Syndrome during Exercise

Sometimes when running or exercising, abnormal pressure develops within a closed space in a leg muscle. Called *exertional compartment syndrome,* this condition causes pain that may feel like shin splints, as well as numbness and possibly weakness in the affected muscle. The abnormal pressure returns to normal once the exercise stops. However, if the pressure becomes excessive, muscles, blood vessels, and nerves may be damaged. The best advice is to listen to your body and stop exercising if you're in pain. If you are continually experiencing pain in the front or back of the lower leg when exercising, a surgeon can surgically release or cut the fascia in the affected compartment. You can also try choosing a different exercise.

a bone deficiency such as osteoporosis (reduced bone density) or osteopenia (reduced bone volume).

Treatment of a stress fracture is similar regardless of where the fracture occurs. First of all, it's critical that you stop participating in any activity that causes pain. Initial treatment includes pain management with Tylenol, ice, and compression with either an ACE bandage or a compression stocking. Navicular stress fractures require six to eight weeks of immobilizing the foot in a cast and not putting any weight on the foot. Metatarsal stress fractures are treated with protected weight bearing in either a CAM walker or a surgical shoe for four to six weeks. Tibial stress fractures may benefit from a brace on the lower leg and foot, although this is not necessary. Calcaneal stress fractures are treated with four to six weeks in either a CAM walking cast for protected weight bearing or a below-knee cast for non–weight bearing. You may be able to continue participating in some activities while recovering from a stress fracture: it's safe to bike or swim with a tibial stress fracture and to swim with a metatarsal stress fracture. However, swimming is not advisable if the fracture involves the navicular or calcaneus.

Any other contributing factors need to be addressed, including nutritional, hormonal, or metabolic imbalances; eating disorders; or abnormal menstrual cycles. For example, a physician may recommend that you take calcium

supplements and multivitamins. On the longer term, you may find it beneficial to use a custom-made orthotic to control the position and mechanics of
the foot. Once the affected bone is free of pain, you can gradually return to
playing a sport.

Broken Bones: Complete Fractures

Complete fractures are a relatively common occurrence in the foot and ankle,
both with exercise and sport and with normal daily living. Broken bones in
the foot account for roughly 10 percent of all fractures in the body. Each bone
in the foot and ankle typically has a different fracture pattern depending on
the location of the bone and how it was injured. The appropriate treatment
depends on various factors. In addition, the causes, symptoms, and treatment
of broken bones differ in children versus adults. Bones break more easily in
a child. Immature bones have open growth plates (areas of cartilage that produce bone cells for growth), and in children, the tendons and ligaments are
stronger than the bones, cartilage, and growth plates. Therefore, a twist or a
turn that may cause a sprained ligament in an adult may cause a bone fracture
in a child. For these reasons, we can't give a detailed discussion in this book
for a break in each bone of the foot and ankle. However, we provide some
general background in case you or your child breaks a foot or ankle bone.

Some of the possible causes of a broken bone include falling from a height,
misstepping off a curb or step, dropping an object on the foot or ankle (blunt
trauma), overusing the foot or ankle in exercise or sports, and sustaining a
high-velocity injury such as in a car or skiing accident. Sometimes fractures
also occur from crushing, bending, twisting, or stubbing injuries. Factors that
increase the risk of a foot or ankle fracture include low bone mineral density,
obesity, occupational demands and requirements, participation in high-impact sports, and peripheral neuropathy (see chapter 10).

Symptoms of a fracture in the foot or ankle usually include redness, bruising, swelling, warmth, pain, and, sometimes, obvious deformity. Frequently,
it is difficult to take more than a few steps on a foot or ankle with a broken
bone, but not always. Some people are able to keep walking even with a
fracture.

Diagnosis of a broken bone in the foot or ankle can be tricky, because a lot of the bones in the foot and ankle overlap on an x-ray, making it hard to see fracture lines in certain areas. The podiatrist may take an x-ray of your opposite foot or ankle to compare the two. In children, open growth plates at the ends of the bones also make it challenging to clearly identify a fracture. If diagnosis is difficult, a podiatrist will order specialized imaging such as an MRI, CT scan, or bone scan.

Treatment for a broken bone in the foot or ankle varies significantly from one bone to another and depends on the location of the break in the particular bone, whether the bone is displaced, whether the break extends into a joint or growth plate, the patient's medical condition, how much the patient walks throughout the course of the day, and whether there is an associated open wound or laceration. Fractures that occur in combination with an open wound require urgent care. Being seen within six hours of the initial injury is important, because in this window of time, a cut may be repaired or sutured, limiting the chance for infection. Most broken bones that are in good alignment and not displaced can be treated with immobilization for four to six weeks. Immobilization can range from wearing a stiff-soled shoe or a CAM walker to a below-the-knee plaster or fiberglass cast with crutches. Broken bones that are in poor alignment or are significantly displaced from their normal position may require surgical repair and realignment.

If you suspect that you or your child has a broken bone in the foot or ankle, go to a podiatrist to have it checked. If a broken bone isn't treated properly, the result may be failure of the bone to heal, longer than normal healing time, healing in an improper position, foot deformity, premature closure of a growth plate, and, if a joint is involved, arthritis.

Shoes for Exercise and Sports

Athletic shoes should be sport-specific, particularly if you participate in a sport for more than three hours per week. For example, don't wear a cross-training shoe if you are a recreational jogger or an elite runner. Buy shoes from a store that specializes in athletic shoes and has a good reputation. Take your old shoes into the store so that the salesperson can assess them for the pattern of wear and recommend an appropriate shoe. Also, it helps the sales-person to know which shoe lines you've used successfully in the past. Wear the socks that you use in the sport when having new shoes fitted. If you have a high-arched, or cavus, foot, look for a shoe that provides cushioning and shock absorption. If you have a flattened arch, or flat foot, find a shoe that provides motion control. Shoe manufacturers make a range of shoes, some of which use a last designed to control excessive pronation (flat feet); these shoes are often referred to as straight last shoes. (A *last* is the overall shape of the shoe; see chapter 3.)

Although it may seem obvious, we recommend that new shoes *not* be worn on race day. Also, pay attention to the condition of your shoes. Even if the shoe and sole don't have obvious signs of wear, the shock-absorbing qual-ity may no longer perform adequately. Running shoes, for example, typically last for 350 to 500 miles.

Chapter 15

Foot Health for People with Diabetes

DIABETES MELLITUS, FREQUENTLY REFERRED to simply as diabetes, is a serious and currently incurable disorder in which the body's cells have difficulty absorbing sugar to use for energy. The sugar accumulates in the blood and may lead to a host of complications such as nerve damage, poor blood circulation, and fragile skin. Diabetes affects over 23 million children and adults—nearly 8 percent of the population—in the United States. New diagnoses of diabetes in adults 20 years and older number at 1.6 million every year, while roughly a quarter of the people with diabetes have not had the condition diagnosed. These statistics, current to 2007, are compiled by the American Diabetes Association.

Although it can't be cured, diabetes can be managed. However, people with diabetes must be vigilant about controlling the diabetes and maintaining their overall health. The health of the lower limbs, and particularly the feet, is critical for reasons that we discuss in this chapter. We first describe diabetes in more detail, then discuss why people with diabetes must pay attention to their feet, and finally outline the preventive measures that people with diabetes can follow to maximize their foot health and lead as full a life as any other person.

What Is Diabetes?

When we eat, our bodies digest the food and convert it into several basic components, one of which is sugar. Sugar enters the bloodstream in the form of glucose, which the body needs for fuel, or energy. To convert glucose into energy, the body uses a hormone called insulin, normally produced by the pancreas. If the pancreas doesn't produce insulin or if the body can't use insulin, the amount of glucose in the blood rises too high. A person with this situation has diabetes. There are two types of diabetes:

- Type 1 diabetes is inherited and used to be called juvenile diabetes, because it is most frequently diagnosed in childhood. With type 1 diabetes, the insulin-producing cells in the pancreas have been destroyed, and therefore they are incapable of producing insulin. People with type 1 diabetes manage the condition through the use of external insulin, which must be administered by injection or with an insulin pump.
- Type 2 diabetes is the more common of the two types and is typically diagnosed in adults. It occurs when the pancreas doesn't produce enough insulin or the body can't use the insulin that is produced (commonly referred to as insulin resistance). Most people with type 2 diabetes manage the condition with oral medication, medical care, diet, and exercise. Many factors predispose a person to developing type 2 diabetes, including age, obesity, and poor dietary habits.

Diabetes, even when it's well managed, increases a person's risk of developing other medical problems. People with unmanaged or poorly managed diabetes—and the accompanying elevated or fluctuating blood sugar over a long period—are at greatest risk. Problems associated with diabetes include damage to major organ systems within the body, such as the skin, nerves, kidneys, eyes, and blood vessels. The immune system becomes impaired, decreasing the body's ability to fight infection. Diabetes can also lead to heart disease and stroke. The longer a person has diabetes, the greater the chance that these problems will occur. However, people who are diagnosed later in life—in their sixties, seventies, or eighties—may not develop further complications, provided that their diabetes is strictly managed.

Why Pay Attention to the Feet?

Diabetes affects the body's blood circulation, so nerves and tissues often don't receive enough blood supply, especially nerves and tissues in the extremities. Damaged nerves reduce sensation in the legs and feet and increase the risk of injuring the skin. Even seemingly minor abrasions can become infected and lead to serious complications because diabetes also compromises the immune system. In addition, nerve and tissue damage can cause the shape and function of the foot to be altered over time. In fact, a complication with the lower extremity is the primary reason for a person with diabetes to be admitted to the hospital. Diabetes is also the leading cause of nontraumatic amputation of the leg.

Blood Circulation

Diabetes tends to cause poor blood circulation to the legs and feet, a condition known as *peripheral vascular disease*. Diabetes in combination with high blood pressure, smoking, or elevated cholesterol and lipids in the blood can lead to a narrowing of the blood vessels. Narrowing of the blood vessels mainly affects the arteries, which are responsible for taking blood away from the heart and delivering it to the peripheral tissues. With poor circulation, the arteries have difficulty delivering oxygen and nutrients to the legs and feet to keep tissues healthy. A lack of adequate blood flow to the feet causes symptoms of pain, cramping in the feet and legs, swelling, redness, dry skin, sores, thickened toe nails, and fatigue. If you have diabetes, you can reduce the chance of developing peripheral vascular disease by exercising regularly and controlling your blood sugar.

Nerves

Consistently elevated blood sugar causes nerve damage, termed *neuropathy*. Nobody yet knows exactly how the nerves are damaged. There are many theories, but the primary cause may be related to poor circulation, which makes it difficult for damaged blood vessels to deliver oxygen and nutrients to the nerves. The risk of nerve damage increases with age and with a longer duration of having diabetes. There are four types of neuropathy: peripheral, autonomic, proximal, and focal. *Peripheral neuropathy* affects the sensory and motor nerves in the hands, arms, feet, and legs. Sensory nerves transmit sensations like pain and temperature, as well as proprioreception (a person's sense of the body's position) and balance back to the brain. Motor nerves control muscles and therefore movement. *Autonomic neuropathy* involves the heart, bladder, lungs, stomach, intestines, sex organs, sweat glands, eyes, and blood vessels. *Proximal neuropathy* causes pain in the thighs, hip, and buttock. *Focal neuropathy,* or mononeuropathy, occurs in a single nerve anywhere in the body and usually has a sudden onset of severe pain and weakness in the area served by the affected nerve.

The foot and lower leg are primarily affected by peripheral neuropathy, in which there is gradual loss of feeling in the arms, hands, legs, and feet. Typically, the loss of feeling occurs in the same areas of both feet and both legs. If you have peripheral neuropathy, you will not feel pain and temperature as well as before, with the obvious consequence of not realizing you've hurt a foot or leg. You may experience a variety of sensations, including numbness, tingling, dull or aching pain, shooting pain, burning, and weakness. When muscles lose nerve function, they become weaker, and they waste away, or atrophy, leading to muscle imbalance, loss of joint stability, joint stiffness, and foot deformity. Foot deformity creates bony prominences that are susceptible to pressure, friction, and shearing forces from wearing shoes, or from a bed, chair, or wheelchair. Along with a loss of sensation, having more pressure points on the foot increases the risk of developing open wounds, or ulcers. Although it sounds drastic, amputation is a common consequence of ulcers on the legs and feet of people with diabetes. We discuss ulcers in more detail later in this chapter, in a section on the skin.

Once peripheral neuropathy develops, there is an increased chance of developing a degenerative condition called Charcot neuroarthropathy, which affects the joints in the foot and ankle by progressively damaging ligaments, cartilage, and bone. The neuroarthropathic disease itself develops slowly, but the bones and joints in the foot can suddenly crumble, fracture, or dislocate. This damage occurs very quickly and often with no more trauma than simply walking around in normal daily activities. When the foot is close to being damaged like this, it becomes red, hot, and swollen, looking like it has an acute infection or cellulitis (inflammation under the skin). If the foot is immediately treated with up to three months of immobilization, its shape and structure can be saved. However, if your foot is in this situation and you continue to put weight on it, the bones will fracture or crumble, and the joints will dislocate, creating significant deformity in the foot. Often, the arch collapses, referred to as a *rocker bottom foot*, and bony prominences form. These prominences are subjected to abnormal and excessive forces, increasing the risk of developing ulcers and infection.

The Skin and Infection

The skin is the body's first line of defense, protecting us from external pressure and preventing bacteria from entering the body. Beneath the skin, blood vessels and nerves provide vital functions to keep the body healthy. Diabetes damages small blood vessels that normally nourish the skin, so the skin often becomes dry and cracked, forming a perfect route for bacteria to enter the body. Once bacteria penetrate to the deeper layers of skin, a superficial infection, called *cellulitis*, may develop. With cellulitis, the skin becomes red, hot, swollen, and tender. Treatment depends on its severity and often includes oral antibiotics, elevation of the affected body part, and compression with an ACE bandage to help control the swelling. Damage to the small blood vessels within the skin may also cause brown spots or scars to form on the feet and legs, called *diabetic dermopathy*. This condition is a cosmetic issue. Fungal infections of the skin and toenails are also more likely to occur in people with diabetes, because of their weakened immune system. (See chapter 6 for information on treating fungal infections.)

A significant skin complication for people with diabetes is the formation of an ulcer. Ulcers are wounds that, on the foot, occur most frequently over bony prominences that are subjected to repetitive, chronic pressure or friction. Wounds can vary in depth from superficial ones that don't even break through the skin to deep ones that extend to the soft tissues of the subcutaneous layer, to muscles, and even to bone. They may or may not appear to be open wounds. For example, both superficial and deep ulcers can occur and be hidden under calluses, corns, or blisters, as illustrated in figure 15.1.

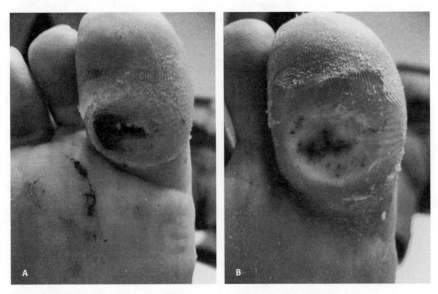

Figure 15.1. (A) A callus with dark red dried blood within is suspicious for an underlying problem. (B) Cutting away the overlying callus reveals an underlying ulcer.

Early identification and proper treatment of an ulcer is critical to ensure that the skin heals properly. The goal is to get the wound to heal as quickly as possible before infection develops. Proper wound care—which should only be done by a podiatrist or other physician—starts with cutting into the ulcer to remove unhealthy tissue and to stimulate bleeding. Blood brings oxygen and nutrients to the ulcer site and promotes the release of other biological agents that are essential for healing. All sources of pressure or friction must be removed, because they will prevent the wound from healing, and worse, can lead to deeper wound penetration and infection. In addition to dealing with the ulcer itself, the podiatrist will evaluate you for abnormalities in the feet resulting in excessive pressure as well as for adequate blood sugar control, nutrition, blood circulation, and sensation in the feet. Problems in any of these areas may require a referral to another specialist, such as a nutritionist, endocrinologist (an expert in hormones and other substances carried by the blood), or vascular surgeon (who assesses and treats problems with blood vessels and circulation).

If ulcers are not treated, infection will likely develop as bacteria invade the skin and soft tissues. Signs of infection include intense redness and possibly red streaks, swelling, warmth, pain, and pus. If you have diabetes and suspect that you may have a foot infection, go to see a podiatrist immediately. Treatment depends on the severity of the infection. Infections that extend to the deeper soft tissues or to bone often require surgical drainage, surgical cutting away of dead or infected tissue, and sometimes amputation. To help fight the infection, a podiatrist will prescribe antibiotics that are targeted at the specific bacteria growing in the wound. The type of bacteria is determined by taking a swab of the affected tissue and culturing the bacteria in a laboratory. The depth and extent of the infection dictates how long you continue to take antibiotics.

Prevention Is the Best Medicine

The best thing you can do as a person with diabetes is take care of yourself and, as much as possible, prevent the disorder from taking its toll on your health. To help you with this prevention, you should have a primary care physician or family doctor, and you may have regular appointments with other specialists, such as an endocrinologist, a podiatrist, and an eye specialist. Ideally, you should see a nutritionist, if not regularly then at least for an initial consultation. There are a few basic actions that you should do without fail: regularly visit your primary care physician to ensure strict control of blood sugar levels, take all medications exactly as prescribed, eat a healthy diet, refrain from smoking, and participate in regular exercise, unless given other instructions from a physician. Exercise improves bone health, promotes circulation, and helps to stabilize blood sugar levels.

Because of the complications for the feet that we outlined earlier, you should be referred to a podiatrist as soon as a diagnosis of diabetes is made. The podiatrist evaluates your medical history and performs a physical examination to develop a foot care program tailored to you. Typically, you should see a podiatrist once a year for an assessment, although some people require more frequent evaluations. If you have or are at particular risk of developing the neurological or vascular complications described earlier, you should go to a podiatrist every two to three months for preventive foot care, including trimming of nails, corns, and calluses. You should also inspect your feet every day to look for changes in the skin, the toenails, or the shape of the foot. Report any abnormalities to your podiatrist or primary care physician. A callus or wart can sometimes conceal a more serious problem, such as an abscess.

If you have diabetes, proper hygiene and skin care are essential. Wash your feet every day with mild soap and water, paying particular attention between the toes. If the web spaces aren't cleaned, dead skin can accumulate, and fungal and bacterial infections may develop and result in ulcers. We don't recommend soaking feet, as this will lead to dry skin, which is more likely to crack and may put you at risk of infection. Moisturize the skin on your feet twice daily, but don't apply lotion between the toes, because this may encourage a fungal infection or athlete's foot. Cut toenails straight across or file them. Avoid cutting deep into the corners of the nail, because of the increased risk of causing an ingrown toenail. If a nail does become ingrown, immediately consult a podiatrist. Feet that are excessively moist from perspiration can benefit from the use of nonmedicated foot powders, but avoid letting the powder build up between the toes. Antiperspirants can also be used for moist feet.

As a person with diabetes, you should always wear shoes when walking. Walking barefoot increases the chance of getting a puncture wound or an object embedded in the foot, either of which can lead to serious infection and even amputation. If you have peripheral neuropathy, wear shoes when swimming—in a lake, a river, or even a swimming pool.

A podiatrist can recommend the most appropriate type of shoe to wear, depending on the shape of your foot and whether you have peripheral neuropathy or poor circulation. Choose shoes made of a breathable, soft material such as natural leather. Avoid shoes made of plastic or other synthetic materials as well as high-heeled shoes because of the abnormal pressure they put on the forefoot and toes. Before putting on a shoe, always check it for objects, prominent seams, or rough areas that could harm the skin. Wear seamless socks with moisture-absorbing capabilities, and protect your feet from extremes of hot and cold. Individuals with poor circulation, loss of feeling in their feet, significant deformity of the foot, or a history of developing ulcers will benefit from wearing therapeutic shoes designed with special features not provided by off-the-shelf footwear.

The Right Shoe: Therapeutic Shoes

Everyone should wear proper shoes, but for people with diabetes, wearing proper shoes is crucial to their health. If you have diabetes and experience particular or recurring problems with your feet, then ask a podiatrist about therapeutic shoes for diabetes. Therapeutic shoes can be considered medical devices. They are specially designed with consideration for the possible repercussions of diabetes, including poor circulation, loss of sensation, joint stiffness, excess strain on the foot, and amputation. As sensation diminishes in the feet, people with diabetes are susceptible to skin injury from repetitive pressing or rubbing of poorly fitting shoes. The goal of a therapeutic shoe is to reduce this repetitive tissue trauma to the foot. In addition to the shoe itself, therapeutic shoes come with accommodative insoles, which are described in more detail in chapter 16. The therapeutic shoe and the accommodative insole together help to reduce injury and improve function.

The U.S. government introduced a Therapeutic Shoe Bill in the early 1990s to focus on ulcer prevention for people with diabetes. This bill stipulates that a person with diabetes can receive partial coverage of the cost of therapeutic shoes if at least one of the following situations applies: prior amputation of part of the foot, a history of developing ulcers or lesions that lead to ulcers, foot deformity, poor circulation, loss of sensation, or neuropathy. In addition to having one of these conditions, a person must be under the comprehensive care of an endocrinologist or a primary care physician. A podiatrist gives the prescription for therapeutic shoes.

There are two types of therapeutic shoe: an extra-depth shoe, which is obtained off-the-shelf according to foot size (figure 15.2), and a custom-made shoe, which is made over a mold of the person's foot (figure 15.3). The custom-made shoe is typically reserved for people whose feet have lost all sensation and are significantly deformed. All therapeutic shoes have similar qualities. The shoe is lightweight and has good shock absorption and a last shape that is compatible with the foot type. The upper of the shoe is breathable to diminish moisture and heat and seamless to avoid rubbing or pressure on the foot. It has a padded tongue, a firm heel counter, and a rocker sole to reduce forefoot pressure. The shoe has additional depth throughout to

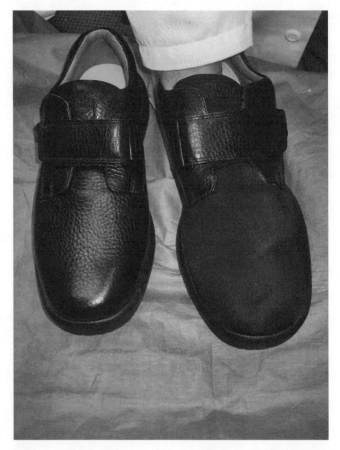

Figure 15.2. Therapeutic shoes such as these are available prefabricated and have heat mold-able inserts to accommodate and offload areas of pressure on the sole of the foot. The shoe on the right has an upper made of an expandable material.

accommodate insoles and modifications to insoles. The sole of the shoe, both the outsole and the midsole, should be the same width as the upper to avoid bulging of the upper with a wider foot. Ideally, the shoelaces or Velcro straps are attached to a piece of leather that is then stitched onto the rest of the shoe. This way, if the foot swells, the soft upper part of the shoe can expand freely without being limited by tight laces or Velcro straps.

Many podiatrists provide a service for patients to buy therapeutic shoes at their office, similar to many ophthalmologists providing eyeglass services.

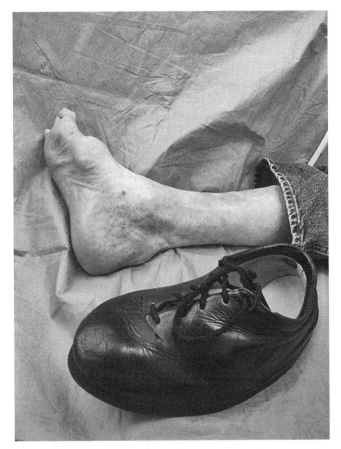

Figure 15.3. This custom-made therapeutic shoe with special accommodative inserts has helped this patient with diabetes to remain free of ulcers for fifteen years, despite significant foot deformity and the presence of neuropathy.

Alternatively, you can buy therapeutic shoes from a specialized shoe store or from a pedorthotist or prosthetist. Techniques to ensure that the shoe fits well are the same as for fitting any shoe. Regularly inspect your therapeutic shoes and insoles for signs of wear and replace them when necessary. The Therapeutic Shoe Bill allows for one new pair of shoes and three pairs of diabetic insoles per year.

Chapter 16

Orthotic Devices to Alleviate
Foot Problems

FOR MANY PEOPLE, shoes alone are not enough to provide adequate support, stability, or comfort. These people may have a foot shape that is poorly supported by off-the-shelf shoes, or they may be recovering from foot surgery. Whatever the reason, a range of insoles, splints, braces, and other devices can be used to provide support, redistribute pressure, and improve overall function of the foot and ankle. Collectively, these products are called orthotics, or orthoses. They can be bought ready-made or they can be custom made for an individual's foot. Throughout the chapters in this book describing foot disorders and other problems, we have frequently noted that an orthotic may be a useful treatment option. In some cases, particularly when a person is a poor candidate for surgery, an orthotic is the only realistic option. This chapter discusses the two basic types of orthotic, a foot orthotic and an ankle–foot orthotic, each of which has specific functions.

Much More than an Insole: Foot Orthotics

Many people think a foot orthotic is simply a fancy insole to provide arch support. In reality, it is a device that can alleviate the symptoms of a foot disorder and restore alignment and function of a foot. If properly designed, an orthotic can also improve muscle and tendon function while supporting the bones of the foot and ankle. Foot orthotics are used to reduce pain, increase stability, provide support, accommodate or correct a deformity or misalignment, minimize stress, absorb shock, and improve balance. This is not simply an arch support! A foot orthotic fits inside your shoe and extends along the bottom of the foot from the back of the heel to just behind the ball. Soft extensions are sometimes added to the top of an orthotic to extend under the ball of the foot or to the ends of the toes, especially if there is pain in the ball.

There are off-the-shelf and custom-made varieties of foot orthotic. The off-the-shelf products are more affordable and are best suited to people with mild symptoms and minimal deformity. They can be modified by a physician as needed. However, if your foot disorder or condition is more severe, then a custom-made foot orthotic is often the better choice, because it will contour perfectly to the bottom of your foot. Custom-made orthotics are made from an impression of your foot, which can be obtained by computer scan, using compressible foam, and most commonly, with a plaster casting of the foot. Computer scans and plaster impressions can be done with the foot weight bearing, partially weight bearing, or non–weight bearing, while compressible foam molds can be done with partial or full weight bearing. A plaster cast allows a physician to make an impression of the foot in the desired position, as shown in figure 16.1.

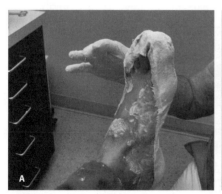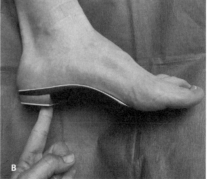

Figure 16.1. (A) A plaster impression is taken while the foot is held in a neutral position. (B) A foot orthotic made from a plaster casting perfectly fits the foot's contours.

The scan, foam impression, or plaster cast is sent to a laboratory, where a reproduction of the foot is made, and an orthotist or a pedorthist makes the orthotic based on the reproduction and a prescription describing the biomechanics of your foot, the range of motion in the foot and ankle, and how active you are or would like to be.

Each of the methods of taking a foot impression offers advantages and disadvantages. Computer scans and foam impressions are clean, fast, and easy to do; however, they allow less control in maintaining the foot in the desired position, so the final orthotic might not be as accurate as it can be when a plaster impression is taken. Plaster casting is preferable for feet with exceptional features, such as an especially high or low arch, or for a very flexible foot that might not stay in position when placed in foam.

The idea behind a custom-made orthotic is to restore a "normal," or neutral, foot position, as we described in chapter 1, and therefore to restore the foot's function. Much of the theory behind today's custom-made orthotics industry is based on the research of the late Dr. Merton Root, who first defined a neutral foot position in the 1970s. It's not always possible, of course, to return a foot to the neutral position, which is evident with the three types of foot orthotic: functional, accommodative, or a combination of functional and accommodative.

A functional orthotic attempts to control and change foot function. These devices are usually made of a rigid material, such as polypropylene, acrylic, or carbon fiber–graphite, that resists abnormal forces. They are very durable and will typically last for five to ten years—though sometimes longer or shorter, depending on the physical use and demand on the orthotic. Functional foot orthotics are frequently used to correct flat or pronated feet.

An accommodative orthotic is used to attenuate shock, redistribute pressure off sore spots or areas with ulcers, and improve balance. These devices are made of soft, compressible materials, such as foam, to decrease pressure and rubbing on the foot, as shown in figure 16.2. An accommodative orthotic makes no attempt to rigidly control foot motion. They are best suited to people with a rigid high-arched foot; a rigid, nonmobile, arthritic flat foot; or painful skin lesions on the feet. In addition, people with poor circulation or loss of feeling in the foot, such as some people with diabetes, can benefit from

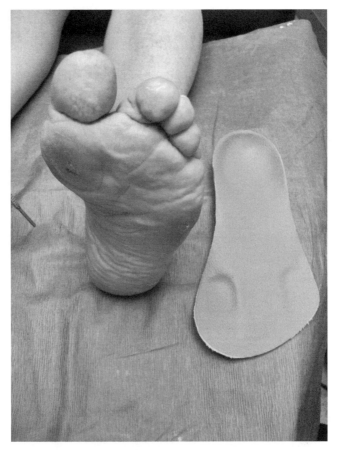

Figure 16.2. This accommodative orthotic has pockets below the first and fifth metatarsal heads to reduce pressure on the painful calluses below those prominent bones.

wearing an accommodative foot orthotic. Because these devices are made from soft materials, they tend to be less durable than functional orthotics and often need to be replaced every one to three years.

A third type of foot orthotic combines both accommodative and functional elements. Typically, these orthotics are made using soft layers reinforced with more rigid materials. These combination orthotics are oc-casionally used by athletes and can also be helpful for people who have a significantly misshapen foot and cannot tolerate the rigidity of a functional foot orthotic.

L-Shaped Braces: Ankle–Foot Orthotics

An ankle–foot orthotic is a brace that encompasses the lower leg, ankle, and foot. The brace is shaped like a large L and typically extends from underneath the toes or ball of the foot along the bottom of the foot, around the heel, behind the ankle, and up the back of the lower leg to below the knee. Some braces wrap around the top of the foot and front of the ankle and are a lace-up variety, and others end below the calf muscle. The shoe keeps the brace on the foot, and Velcro straps wrap around the leg either above the ankle or below the knee to keep the brace snug on the leg. If joints higher up the limb also need support, the brace will include the knee and hip as well. Most of these braces fit inside the shoe.

An ankle–foot orthotic has many functions. It can control motion, provide stability, decrease pain, and transfer weight to another area. It can also correct flexible deformities while preventing the deformity from becoming any worse. Last, an ankle–foot orthotic reduces the energy it takes for you to walk by helping to increase the efficiency of your gait and by minimizing the risk of falling. These braces are commonly used to help people who have a disorder that creates muscle weakness, including stroke, spinal cord injury, muscular dystrophy, cerebral palsy, multiple sclerosis, and nerve entrapment syndromes of the leg. An ankle–foot orthotic may also be used to immobilize and take weight off the foot and ankle in cases of bone fracture, rigid and painful arthritis, Charcot neuroarthropathy, avascular necrosis, tendinitis and tendinosis, and peripheral neuropathy. In addition, individuals with a severe deformity who are unable to undergo surgery can benefit from using this type of orthotic.

An ankle–foot orthotic can be bought off-the-shelf or it can be custom made to fit your specific needs, such as the Arizona and Richie braces shown in figure 16.3. Typically, braces are made of a lightweight material such as a polypropylene-based plastic. Some are made with metal, leather, synthetic fabrics, or any combination of these materials. The brace is usually covered or lined with soft padding to minimize pressure and rubbing on the skin. Depending on the situation and exact function required of an ankle–foot orthotic, it can be rigid or flexible. A rigid, or static, brace, as its name implies,

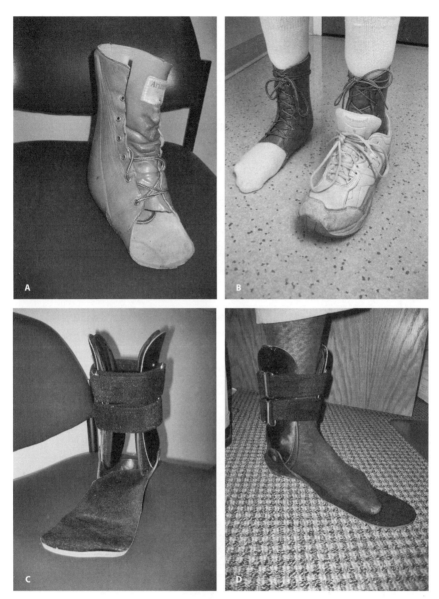

Figure 16.3. Two types of custom-made ankle–foot orthotics: (A) An Arizona brace. (B) An Arizona brace, which fits inside the shoe, controls up and down as well as in and out motion of the foot. (C) A Richie brace. (D) A Richie brace also fits inside the shoe, controlling in and out motion of the foot while allowing up and down motion at the ankle.

doesn't have any moving parts. It is used to support a weakened or paralyzed part of the body. A flexible, or dynamic, brace has hinged joints and is used to help the ankle joint move. The hinged joints of a flexible brace, which is usually constructed of metal, can be designed both to help the ankle move as it's supposed to and to limit undesired movements. For example, if you have trouble lifting your foot toward the shin (dorsiflexion), you can wear a brace to help with this action. A brace could also be used to limit downward motion of the ankle (plantarflexion) or to hold the foot in a corrected position so that it doesn't slap hard against the ground or cause you to trip over the toes when walking.

Resources

The following organizations and web sites provide reliable information about foot problems and their treatment.

American Academy of Podiatric Sports Medicine, www.aapsm.org

American Association for Women Podiatrists, www.americanwomen podiatrists.com

American Board of Podiatric Surgery (may soon become the American Board of Foot and Ankle Surgeons), www.abps.org

American College of Foot and Ankle Surgeons, www.acfas.org

American Diabetes Association, www.diabetes.org

American Podiatric Medical Association, www.apma.org

eMedicine medical reference, emedicine.medscape.com

Foot Health Facts, www.foothealthfacts.org

Mayo Clinic medical information, www.mayoclinic.com

Index

walking, 159, 160, 162; tone of, 119; weakness of, 49, 53, 130. *See also* calf muscles; neuromuscular conditions; paralytic muscle diseases

muscular dystrophy, 52, 161, 202

musculoskeletal examination, 24

navicular bone, 5, 6, 130, 163, 165; and stress fractures, 181, 182, 183

nerve conduction studies, 116

nerve entrapment syndromes, 48, 52–53, 202

nerves: and Achilles tendon rupture, 149; anatomy of, 113–14; Baxter's, 105, 112; and bunions, 92; compressed, 115, 120; and diabetes, 187, 188, 189–90; disorders of, 20; intermetatarsal, 121; irritation of, 31; in lower back, 115–17; peroneal, 123–26; sural, 123, 125, 126; syndromes of, 113–27; tibial, 119

neurectomy, 127

neuritis, 31

neurological examination, 24

neurologists, 21

neurolysis, 123

neuromuscular conditions, 48, 52, 53, 54, 98, 157, 160–61

neuropathy, 60, 189–90. *See also* peripheral neuropathy

neutral position, 8, 15, 16, 35

nevus, 72, 73, 75

nicotine, 69

obesity, 48, 130, 137, 184

oncologists, 21

onychomycosis, 87–89

orthotics, 23, 26, 27, 198–204; and accessory navicular syndrome, 163; and ankle equinus, 42; ankle-foot, 49–50, 162, 202–4; and brachymetatarsia, 169; and dancer's tendonitis, 147; and flat feet, 49; and Haglund's deformity, 109; and hammertoes, 99; and high-arched feet, 53;

and metatarsalgia, 101; and metatarsus adductus, 43, 157; and nerve entrapment syndromes, 126; and osteoarthritis, 132; and peroneal tendons, 144; and plantar fasciitis, 107, 108; and predislocation syndrome, 103; and rheumatoid arthritis, 136; and sesamoid injury, 175; and shin splints, 179; and tarsal coalition, 164; and tarsal tunnel syndrome, 120; and toe walking, 162; and varus and valgus conditions, 40

osteoarthritis, 41, 52, 53, 128–33

osteochondroma, 84, 85–86

osteochondrosis, 165–67

osteopenia, 183

osteoporosis, 181, 182, 183

os tibiale externum, 162

os trigonum bone, 146, 147, 180

os trigonum syndrome, 146

out-toe position (abductus), 5, 11, 13, 15, 43, 153, 158–59

overpronation, 47, 110, 167, 177

pain: and accessory navicular syndrome, 162–63; and Achilles tendon rupture, 148; and bunions, 92, 93; in calf, 126; and common peroneal nerve, 124; and corns and calluses, 62–63; and dancer's tendonitis, 146; and deep peroneal nerve, 126; and flat feet, 49, 50; and Freiberg infraction, 166; and gout, 137, 138; and hammertoes, 98; and high-arched feet, 53; and metatarsalgia, 100–101; and Morton's neuroma, 121, 122; and nerve entrapment syndromes, 127; and osteoarthritis, 131–32; and peripheral neuropathy, 117, 118; and peroneal tendons, 143; and plantar fasciitis, 105–6, 107; and predislocation syndrome, 101–2, 103; and rheumatoid arthritis, 135, 136; and stress fractures, 182, 183; and superficial peroneal nerve, 125–26; and sural nerve, 126; and tarsal coalition, 164;